Inside—Find the Answers to These Questions and More

- ☑ Can calcium supplements relieve all major PMS symptoms? (See page 62.)

- ☑ What type of calcium should I take and how much? (See page 72.)

- ☑ How does chasteberry help PMS? (See page 80.)

- ☑ Does ginkgo help reduce PMS-related fluid retention and breast tenderness? (See page 104.)

- ☑ What is evening primrose oil and can it help PMS? (See page 84.)

- ☑ Can kava help reduce my anxiety during PMS? (See page 120.)

- ☑ Which PMS symptoms can vitamin E relieve? (See page 96.)

- ☑ Is vitamin B_6 really effective for PMS? (See page 100.)

- ☑ Are there other conditions that might be mistaken for PMS? (See page 12.)

- ☑ Do I have any alternative to Prozac for my PMS depression? (See page 115.)

THE NATURAL PHARMACIST™ Library

Natural Health Bible
Your Complete Guide to Illnesses and
Their Natural Remedies
Your Complete Guide to Herbs
Your Complete Guide to Vitamins and Supplements
Feverfew and Migraines
Heart Disease Prevention
Kava and Anxiety
Arthritis
Colds and Flus
Diabetes
Garlic and Cholesterol
Ginkgo and Memory
Menopause
PMS
Reducing Cancer Risk
Saw Palmetto and the Prostate
St. John's Wort and Depression
Preventing Osteoporosis with Ipriflavone

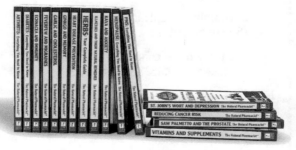

Visit us online at www.TNP.com

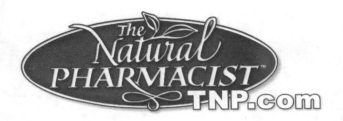

Everything You Need to Know About

PMS

Helen J. Batchelder

Series Editors

Steven Bratman, M.D.

David Kroll, Ph.D.

Prima
HEALTH

A DIVISION OF PRIMA PUBLISHING

Visit us online at www.TNP.com

© 1999, 2000 BY PRIMA PUBLISHING

Warning—Disclaimer

Pseudonyms are used throughout to protect the privacy of individuals involved.

PRIMA HEALTH and colophon are trademarks of Prima Communications, Inc.

THE NATURAL PHARMACIST™ is a trademark of Prima Communications, Inc.

Illustrations © Prima Publishing. All rights reserved. Illustrations by Helene D. Stevens and Gale Mueller.

All products mentioned in this book are trademarks of their respective companies.

Library of Congress Cataloging-in-Publication Data

Batchelder, Helen J.
    PMS / Helen J. Batchelder.
        p.   cm.—(The natural pharmacist)
    Includes bibliographical references and index.
    ISBN 0-7615-1615-8
    1. Premenstrual syndrome—Popular works.   2. Premenstrual syndrome—
Alternative treatment—Popular works.   I. Title.   II. Series.
RG165.B38   1999
618.1'72—dc21   98-49608
                                                                                                    CIP

00 01 02 HH 10 9 8 7 6 5 4
Printed in the United States of America

Visit us online at www.TNP.com

Contents

What Makes This Book Different?

The interest in natural medicine has never been greater. According to the National Association of Chain Drug Stores, 65 million Americans are using natural supplements, and the number is growing! Yet, it is hard for the consumer to find trustworthy sources for balanced information about this emerging field. Why? Frankly, natural medicine has had a checkered history. From snake oil potions sold at the turn of the century to those books, magazines, and product catalogs that hype miracle cures today, this is a field where exaggerated claims have been the norm. Proponents of natural medicine have tended to abuse science, treating it more as a marketing tool than a means of discovering the truth.

But there is truth to be found. Studies of vitamins, minerals, and other food supplements have been with us since these nutritional substances were first discovered, and the level and quality of this science has grown dramatically in the last 20 years. Herbal medicine has been neglected in the United States, but in Europe, this, the oldest of all healing arts, has been the subject of tremendous and ongoing scientific interest.

At present, for a number of herbs and supplements, it is possible to give reasonably scientific answers to the questions: How well does this work? How safe is it? What types of conditions is it best used for?

THE NATURAL PHARMACIST series is designed to cut through the hype and tell you what we know and what we don't know about popular natural treatments. These books are more conservative than any others available, more honest about the weaknesses of natural approaches, more fair in their comparisons of natural and conventional treatments. You won't find any miracle cures here, but you will discover useful options that can help you become healthier.

Why Choose Natural Treatments?

Although the science behind natural medicine continues to grow, this is still a much less scientifically validated field than conventional medicine. You might ask, "Why should I resort to an herb that is only partly proven, when I could take a drug with solid science behind it?" There are at least three good reasons to consider natural alternatives.

First, some herbs and supplements offer benefits that are not matched by any conventional drug. Vitamin E is a good example. It appears to help prevent prostate cancer, a benefit that no standard medication can claim.

Another example is the herb milk thistle. Studies strongly suggest that this herb can protect the liver from injury. There is no pill or tablet your doctor can prescribe to do the same.

Even if the science behind some of these treatments is less than perfect, when the risks are low and the possible benefit high, a natural treatment may be worth trying. It is a little-known fact that for many conventional treatments the science is less than perfect as well, and physicians must balance uncertain benefits against incompletely under-stood risks.

A second reason to consider natural therapies is that some may offer benefits comparable to those of drugs with fewer side effects. The herb St. John's wort is a good exam-ple. Reasonably strong scientific evidence suggests that this herb is an effective treatment for mild to moderate depres-sion, while producing fewer side effects on average than conventional medications. Saw palmetto for benign en-largement of the prostate, ginkgo for relieving symptoms and perhaps slowing the progression of Alzheimer's disease, and glucosamine for osteoarthritis are other examples. This is not to say that herbs and supplements are completely harmless—they're not—but for most the level of risk is quite low.

Finally, there is a philosophical point to consider. For many people, it "feels" better to use a treatment that comes from nature instead of from a laboratory. Just as you might rather wear all-cotton clothing than polyester, or look at a mountain landscape rather than the skyscrapers of a downtown city, natural treatments may simply feel more compatible with your view of life. We can quibble endlessly about just what "natural" means and whether a certain treatment is "actually" natural or not, but such ar-guments are beside the point. The difference is in the feel-ing, and feelings matter. In fact, having a good feeling about taking an herb may lead you to use it more consis-tently than you would a prescription drug.

Of course, at times synthetic drugs may be necessary and even lifesaving. But on many other occasions it may be quite reasonable to turn to an herb or supplement instead of a drug.

To make good decisions you need good information. Unfortunately, while hundreds of books on alternative medicine are published every year, many are highly mis-leading. The phrase "studies prove" is often used when the studies in question are so small or so badly conducted that they prove nothing at all. You may even find that the "data" from other books comes from studies with petri dishes and not real people!

You can't even assume that books written by well-known authors are scientifically sound. Many of these authors rely on secondary writers, leading to a game of "telephone," where misconceptions are passed around from book to book. And there's a strong tendency to exaggerate the power of natural remedies, whitewashing them with selective reporting.

THE NATURAL PHARMACIST series gives you the balanced information you need to make informed decisions about your health needs. Setting a new, high standard of accuracy and objectivity, these books take a realistic look at the herbs and supplements you read about in the news. You will encounter both favorable and unfavorable studies in these pages and will learn about both the benefits and the risks of natural treatments.

THE NATURAL PHARMACIST series is the source you can trust.

Steven Bratman, M.D.
David Kroll, Ph.D.

Introduction

If you are one of the many women who suffer from premenstrual syndrome (PMS), you are surely familiar with the disturbing effects it has on both your physical and emotional well-being. For a few weeks each month, you may endure sudden mood swings, depression, anxiety, weight gain, headaches, and a variety of physical and emotional discomforts. But there is something else you must also experience and it may seem equally as disturbing: PMS is a disorder that is so widely misunderstood that many people simply refuse to acknowledge its existence.

You may have discovered that your family and coworkers regard it as something you should be able to control. Your employer's reaction to PMS may be to tell you to "just snap out of it." PMS has even become the subject of countless jokes. But, as you know, PMS is no laughing matter.

Premenstrual syndrome is a real medical disorder, one with physical causes and one that can have drastic effects on your everyday life. If you are like many women, PMS can be a private torture that you suffer with little or no support from family, friends, and coworkers. It is difficult to imagine these same people joking about other disorders, such as diabetes, or believing that diabetes is all in the minds of those who suffer from it. Still, the misconceptions about PMS persist.

The Natural Pharmacist Guide to PMS will give you the facts about this puzzling disorder: what might cause it, how PMS relates to your monthly cycle, modern medicine's conventional treatments for PMS, and up-to-date scientific evidence about the herbal products and supplements that can provide real relief for the upsetting effects of PMS.

While I'll tell you about the conventional pharmaceuticals used to treat PMS, how well you can expect them to work, and what side effects they produce, my emphasis will be on the natural and supplementary treatments. Women around the world are discovering that these therapies not only ease many of the symptoms of PMS, but are also relatively safe and free of bothersome side effects.

This book will tell you about the latest and most exciting development in PMS research: a recent large scientific study that strongly suggests ordinary calcium supplements may be able to relieve virtually all of the core symptoms of PMS. Other supplements may also be able to help with your PMS, and I'll provide the pros and cons of these: vitamin E, magnesium, and multivitamin/mineral supplements.

I'll also tell you about the promise of safe herbal treatments, such as evening primrose oil and its success in treating the PMS breast tenderness and pain known as cyclic mastalgia. Other herbs that may also provide relief for various symptoms include chasteberry, *Ginkgo biloba,* black cohosh, St. John's wort, kava, and feverfew. But most important of all, I'll tell you about all these things in a clear and unbiased manner. You'll discover the truth about both the conventional and natural treatments for PMS: what scientific research has shown and what it has failed to show. *The Natural Pharmacist Guide to PMS* will give you the most practical and effective ways to treat your PMS, all in a way that you will find honest, straightforward, and easy to understand.

CHAPTER

ONE

What Is PMS?

I'm so tired of this roller coaster," Sarah said. "By the time I begin my period, I feel like I'm crawling out of a deep, dark hole. I look back just a day or two and it's hard to believe it was all happening to me—those headaches, the screaming and crying. My poor husband. He must think I'm crazy. There *must* be some way out of this cycle!"

Does this sound familiar? Sarah is 35—a wife, a mother, a Sunday school teacher, and a chef. Sarah's menstrual cycle means a monthly trip through her own personal nightmare called PMS, short for *premenstrual syndrome*. The entire process makes her feel completely out of control, and "less like a woman, less like a human being, and more like a child's toy being pulled around by Godzilla."

Sarah's husband often tells her that she's being too hard on herself, and that she really isn't *that* bad. But he'll be the first to admit that she's pretty tough to take when she's "that way."

For Sarah, PMS is no joke. It's not a funny story about some hormone-crazed woman on a rampage. It's a part of her life that is disrupting her family, her work, and who she wants to be.

Sarah's story is not unique. For her and many other women, PMS is all too real. What *is* PMS? What causes it? Why does it affect some women and not others? And why,

PMS is a recurrent disorder that disrupts the emotional and physical aspects of many women's lives for up to 2 weeks out of every month.

after countless visits to the doctor, rounds of prescription medications, and even a trip or two to a therapist, is Sarah's PMS still raging out of control?

The truth about PMS is that we don't know exactly what causes it. In fact, researchers are not even sure why this condition affects some women so severely and doesn't affect others at all. At this time, there is no known cure for PMS.

The good news about PMS is that while we have no magic pill to cure it, you can find help through many effective treatments. There are various medications that can significantly reduce symptoms; however, they all cause side effects, which may be severe. Another option is to try herbal or nutritional remedies that appear to be nearly side-effect free. Impressive evidence tells us that the common supplement calcium, when used properly, can significantly reduce all major PMS symptoms. Other notable options include evening primrose oil and the herb chasteberry. This book will tell you everything you need to know about how to feel better and avoid the frustrating, disruptive, and unpleasant symptoms of PMS.

Why Am I Like This?

PMS stands for *premenstrual syndrome.* It is a recurrent disorder that disrupts the emotional and physical aspects of many women's lives for up to 2 weeks out of every month. Its symptoms can range in intensity from mild to incapacitating. The most common symptoms are sudden mood swings, weight gain, breast pain, irritability, anxiety, and, frequently, a sense of feeling out of control.

An estimated 30 to 40% of women between the ages of 25 and 50 experience mild to moderate symptoms of premenstrual syndrome. The onset of PMS typically follows *menarche* (first menstruation), either by itself or sometimes triggered by a "shock" to the *endocrine* system (the body's hormonal system), such as childbirth, hysterectomy, tubal ligation, or going on or off birth control pills. Heredity appears to play a role in PMS, although specific symptoms may differ from mother to daughter and sister to sister.

PMS affects 30 to 40% of women between the ages of 25 and 50.

Symptoms of PMS

There's no simple way to diagnose PMS. There's no blood test, scan, or examination that will demonstrate conclusively that you are suffering from this condition. While the symptoms will point you in the right direction, what will provide the real proof is *how* and *when* the symptoms appear (and disappear) during your monthly cycle. As I mentioned earlier, the symptoms of PMS occur during the 2 weeks prior to the beginning of your period and disappear with menstruation. Proper diagnosis and treatment depend on finding the relationship between your menstrual cycle and your symptoms.

The symptoms of PMS vary from woman to woman. There are literally *hundreds* of different symptoms, but most women with PMS will experience only a handful of them. The intensity of symptoms not only varies from woman to woman, but also within the same woman from month to month. The symptoms of PMS affect both the emotional and the physical aspects of a woman's well-being.

Emotional Symptoms of PMS

The emotional symptoms of PMS tend to be changes, sometimes sudden, in mood and temperament, which may diminish feelings of satisfaction, contentment, and self-worth. Some women find that the emotional ups and

The symptoms of PMS affect both the emotional and the physical aspects of a woman's well-being.

downs make them feel out of control: sad one day, angry the next. Depression, listlessness, and apathy are also frequently reported. You may lose the desire to engage in normal activities, whether gardening, dating, or simply taking a shower.

You may also feel fatigue. When the alarm goes off in the morning, getting out of bed may seem almost more than you can manage. Knowing that you have to get dressed and head into the

office to face piles of work might bring about feelings of hopelessness and despair. This lack of energy touches every part of your life—your marriage, your children, your job. Life in general can feel like an overwhelming burden.

Irritability is another common symptom. You may even experience a temper you never knew you had, and may respond to words or situations that never bothered

Irene's Story

As a second-grade teacher, Irene's mood swings due to PMS caused her some problems. "During that time of the month," Irene said, "Trying to remain calm and collected can be a real challenge, especially on those days when students act up. One thing's for certain when you're a teacher, you need to stay in control, and that's easier said than done when your PMS is putting you through an emotional wringer."

Because of the nature of her work, Irene was unable to rely on a sedative to keep her calm. A coworker told Irene about how much calcium had helped her maintain her composure when she suffered from mood swings. Next month, Irene was delighted at how much better she felt. "I still know PMS when it strikes, but I don't feel at the mercy of my emotions anymore." Irene is one of many who are finding natural substances beneficial for alleviating PMS. Although stories like this one always sound very encouraging, we really need proper double-blind studies to be assured of a treatment's effectiveness. We'll review some of the research on calcium in chapter 5.

---

you before. Off-color jokes, a toothpaste tube with its top left off, or a missing pen—anything might set you off. Anger arises quickly and disappears just as rapidly. However, friends, family, and coworkers may not be as quick to forget these episodes as you are.

Paranoia and anxiety can also be a part of PMS. Paranoia can make a compliment seem like an insult. You might feel like withdrawing from or avoiding social interactions. Anxiety can mean anything from nervousness to full-blown panic attacks. Breathlessness, shaky hands, rapid heartbeat, and worry can all be part of this scenario. As many women have discovered, this kind of emotional upheaval can become so disturbing that it can jeopardize your relationships, family, and career. (For more information on anxiety in general, see *The Natural Pharmacist Guide to Kava and Anxiety*.)

The emotional upheaval caused by PMS can be serious enough to jeopardize your relationships, family, and career.

To sum up, some of the emotional symptoms you might experience include:

- Sudden mood swings
- Feeling out of control
- Weepiness
- Depression
- Listlessness
- Apathy
- Fatigue
- Irritability
- Bursts of uncontrolled anger
- Paranoia
- Anxiety or panic attacks

If you find yourself experiencing such turmoil before your menstrual cycle, take heart. Many of these symptoms may respond particularly well to remedies that are both safe and natural. For example, calcium, chasteberry (vitex), and kava may relieve symptoms of irritability and depression. We'll tell you more about these treatments in chapters 5, 6, and 10.

Physical Symptoms of PMS

Many physical symptoms of PMS are caused by fluid retention. One of the most apparent is weight gain. Even with mild to moderate PMS, some women report an increase of 5 to 8 pounds during this part of their monthly cycle. Weight gain is almost always accompanied by uncomfortable abdominal bloating. If you are experiencing this, you may feel that your lower abdomen bulges out and is tight to the touch. Your clothes may not fit as well during your 2 weeks of PMS, and you may become self-conscious about your appearance. To add to the misery, either constipation or diarrhea may occur as well.

"I hate the time right before my period," Mary says. "I break out my PMS wardrobe: looser clothes that I can wear without feeling like I'm about to split the seams. Too bad the clothes can't get rid of the awful feeling of being so bloated!"

During PMS, your breasts also may become enlarged and tender, even painful. This symptom, which doctors call *mastalgia,* is one of the most common complaints of PMS. Fluid retention can also be experienced as swollen fingers, ankles, and feet. This could easily make everyday tasks, such as buttoning your blouse or typing on the computer, seem nearly impossible. Often, swollen fingers can affect manual dexterity to such a degree that you get the PMS "dropsies"—a glass of milk slips out of your hand or the handle of a frying pan just seems to fall away.

PMS can also affect your appetite. The thought, sight, or smell of food might make you ravenous. Many women feel an urge to eat foods that are either particularly sweet or very salty, such as potato chips or chocolate bars. For others, such cravings might be for a thick cut of prime rib or a mound of steaming lasagna. Some researchers have suggested that weight gain and bloating may be the result of compulsive eating. However, since both weight gain and bloating occur even when women don't overeat, such a theory has been discounted.

You might also suffer from PMS headaches. Comparable to migraines, such headaches can last as long as 5 days. Their effects can be incapacitating. For example, when

Amy's PMS headaches hit her, as they usually did each month, she would swallow a dose of Advil and retreat back to bed to try to sleep until they let up. She used up a sizable amount of sick leave and bid adieu to many of her weekend plans, but she didn't feel she had much choice when her head started pounding. (For more information on migraines, see *The Natural Pharmacist Guide to Feverfew and Migraines.*)

PMS produces other symptoms too. Your joints might become so stiff that it hurts to stay in one position for very long, or your skin may seem to crawl with painful coldness. Your desire for sex may increase or decrease, creating a sense of confusion for your partner and guilt for you. Other symptoms include lower back pain and the unusual sensation known as "restless legs."

To briefly recap, some of the common physical symptoms of PMS are

- Weight gain
- Abdominal bloating accompanied by either diarrhea or constipation
- Enlarged and painful breasts
- Fluid retention causing swollen fingers, ankles, or feet
- The "dropsies"
- Compulsive eating and cravings for salty or sweet foods
- Headaches
- Stiff joints
- Changes in sexual desire
- Lower back pain
- "Restless legs"

A number of natural products are used to help treat many of these symptoms. Both calcium and chasteberry (vitex) are among those most frequently used. Chasteberry and evening primrose are both helpful for easing the symptoms of painfully swollen breasts, while ginkgo may help all symptoms of fluid retention. For more information about these natural treatments, see chapters 5 through 9.

A Warning About Something More Serious: PDD

Some women experience a form of PMS so severe that it has been given another name: *premenstrual dysphoric disorder* (PDD). PMS is distressing, disruptive, interfering, and annoying, but the symptoms are mild to moderate in scope. PDD symptoms are worse and much more severe. The American Psychiatric Association (APA) is very clear in distinguishing between PMS and PDD.

According to the APA, a woman must experience 5 of the following 11 symptoms, during the last 2 weeks of two consecutive menstrual cycles for her condition to be diagnosed as PDD. Of these five symptoms, depressed mood, anxiety, irritability, or emotional instability must be included.

1. Depressed mood
2. Anxiety
3. Emotional instability
4. Irritability
5. Disinterest, or decreased interest, in usual activities
6. Difficulty concentrating
7. Decrease in, or lack of, energy
8. Undereating, overeating, or food cravings
9. Inability to sleep or excessive sleeping
10. Feeling overwhelmed
11. Physical discomforts, including breast tenderness, headache, and others associated with PMS

If you suffer from these symptoms during the first 2 weeks of the menstrual cycle, this tends to indicate some other underlying condition.

Although women with PMS *may* experience these symptoms, the diagnosing factor is the *severity* of the symptoms. PDD symptoms are likely to get worse as a woman gets older. Typically appearing in a woman's late 20s, the devastating effects of PDD may ruin jobs and relationships by the time she reaches the age of 30.

What's important to know about PDD is that it urgently needs treatment. If you suspect that you are suffering from premenstrual dysphoric disorder, it is important that you see your physician as soon as possible.

Relief from the Symptoms of PMS

The symptoms of PMS are almost always relieved by one simple event: *menstruation*. Women with painful, enlarged breasts often report feeling better in as little as 2 hours after they get their periods. Weight gain, bloating, headaches—all seem to vanish quickly as a feeling of calm ensues.

The symptoms of PMS are almost always relieved by one simple event: *menstruation*.

However, this relief has a few catches. Obviously, you can not menstruate constantly (nor would you want to). And of course, when your period is over, the cycle begins again, repeating itself (and PMS) until the onset of menopause.

Besides menstruation and menopause, you can try other, more reasonable means of relief for these uncomfortable and disturbing symptoms. As we've mentioned, treatments include herbal remedies, dietary supplements, and even exercise. In later chapters, we'll tell you about various natural treatments for PMS, such as calcium, evening primrose oil, chasteberry, ginkgo, magnesium, vitamin B_6, and dong quai, and how they may help you relieve PMS pain, fluid retention, and other symptoms.

Coping with PMS: What You Can Do for Yourself

A woman with PMS goes to her doctor expecting results. No different from anyone else seeking medical care, she's expecting her doctor to look at her symptoms, diagnose her problem, and administer the miracle medication or state-of-the-art treatment. Afterwards, all of her symptoms will disappear. End of story.

Unfortunately, getting treatment for PMS (and many other conditions) is neither this simple nor this satisfying. Although we have no cure for PMS, treatments are available that can help you feel more like your normal self. To find the right ones, however, you will have to become involved in your own care. Whether you are dealing with conventional medicine or some of the natural approaches discussed in this book, coping with your PMS will take both effort and determination.

First, don't be afraid to call your doctor and say, "I think I have PMS. Can we check it out?" Don't let friends, family, or colleagues belittle PMS as a behavior problem. Next, know that the best chance to ensure a positive experience with your doctor is to be very specific about your symptoms and about what you hope to accomplish by consulting him or her. You can be more candid about how the symptoms affect you if you gather information before your visit. Before you see your physician, keep a diary of your PMS symptoms, including when and how each symptom appears during your monthly cycle. (For more information about a PMS diary, see chapter 2.)

Do your homework: Consider all your possible treatment options. If you're unhappy with the side effects of conventional medications, ask your doctor whether he or she knows about the effects of vitamins or herbal supplements on PMS. Discuss how herbal treatments and nutritional supplements have been shown to provide relief for many PMS symptoms. The options discussed in this book are a good starting point.

Disorders with Similar Symptoms

PMS has hundreds of symptoms, many of which are also common in numerous other conditions. It is important, then, to see your doctor to rule out other disorders, some of which can mimic, be mistaken for, or even be masked by PMS.

Hypothyroidism

Hypothyroidism is a condition in which the thyroid gland either stops producing or doesn't produce enough thyroid hormone, a substance your body depends on for regulating metabolism. When the thyroid malfunctions, you may experience such symptoms as weight gain, headaches, fatigue, depression, sensitivity to cold, and abnormal periods.

Herbal treatments and nutritional supplements have been shown to provide relief for many PMS symptoms.

If you suffer from most of these symptoms during all phases of your menstrual cycle, I recommend that you consult with your physician immediately. Most forms of hypothyroidism require hormone treatment.

Depression

Depression is more common than most people realize. At least one person in six experiences a serious, or "major," depressive episode at some time in life. Depression is a mood disorder that can, in most cases, be effectively treated. If you suffer from depression, please seek medical help.

An individual is considered to be suffering from depression if she experiences five or more of the following symptoms:

1. Poor appetite and weight loss, or increased appetite and weight gain
2. Inability to fall asleep or to stay asleep (insomnia), or prolonged or excessive sleep (hypersomnia)
3. Hyperactivity or inactivity
4. Loss of interest or pleasure, or noticeable reduction of interest, in sex
5. Fatigue, loss of energy
6. Feelings of worthlessness, self-reproach, or feeling guilty without cause
7. Diminished ability to concentrate
8. Recurrent thoughts of death or suicide

(For more information on depression, see *The Natural Pharmacist Guide to St. John's Wort and Depression.*)

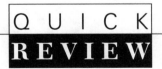

QUICK REVIEW

- The truth about PMS is that its exact cause is not yet known. In fact, researchers are not even sure why some women are so severely affected by it and others are not affected at all. At this time, PMS has no known cure.

- PMS is a recurrent disorder that disrupts the emotional and physical aspects of women's lives for up to 2 weeks out of every month. It affects 30 to 40% of women between the ages of 25 and 50.

- Several nearly side-effect–free natural treatments are available for PMS, particularly the mineral calcium, as well as evening primrose oil, chasteberry (vitex), and ginkgo.
- The symptoms of PMS occur during the 2 weeks prior to the beginning of your period and disappear with menstruation.
- PMS can affect both the emotional and physical well-being of women. Common symptoms include sudden mood swings, weight gain, irritability, anxiety, and frequently a sense of being out of control.
- A medical diagnosis for your PMS will rule out other disorders with similar symptoms such as hypothyroidism and depression.

CHAPTER
T W O

Understanding Your Monthly Cycle

T he menstrual cycle is a monthly process that is governed by a complex interaction of hormones. To comprehend the "hows" and "whys" of PMS, having a basic understanding of how your hormones work is important. This chapter will tell you what we know— and what we don't know—about this complex and fundamental process. But if you'd rather get straight to finding out how natural treatments might provide relief for PMS symptoms, you can skip ahead to chapter 5.

The Endocrine System

Your body's endocrine system is a collection of glands and tissues that produce hormones, which are released, or *secreted*, into the bloodstream and transported to various parts of the body. The word *hormone* is derived from a Greek root that means "to arouse." This is precisely what hormones do—arouse other cells to action.

Once they have reached their destinations, hormones stimulate organs and tissues to affect a variety of actions. Metabolism, growth, and sexual function are just a few of the processes that are controlled by the hormones your endocrine system produces. The entire process is so beautifully interwoven that it is a virtual symphony of chemical responses and interactions.

The Glands of the Endocrine System

The endocrine system includes a variety of glands (see figure 1). Each secretes its own hormones and each makes a vital contribution to help maintain your body's equilibrium and keep it functioning properly. The major glands in your body that play a role in PMS are the

- Hypothalamus
- Pituitary
- Thyroid
- Parathyroid
- Adrenals
- Ovaries

The hypothalamus is a cherry-size bit of brain tissue that monitors the levels of numerous substances in the bloodstream. When it detects that too much or too little of a hormone is present, it sends information to the pituitary gland, which in turn instructs various other glands to increase or decrease hormone production, depending on which is needed.

Virtually all the systems of your body are affected by the hormones controlled by the hypothalamus and the pituitary gland. To function properly, your immune system, digestive system, cardiovascular system, and nervous system all rely on these hormones. Among the many physical processes dependent on hormones are heart rate, blood pressure, metabolism, and the absorption of calcium from the diet.

The hypothalamus also plays a key role in regulating the cyclic and hormonal changes of the menstrual cycle. One of

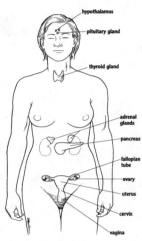

Figure 1. *The endocrine system*

the ways it does so is by producing *gonadotropin-releasing hormone* (GnRH). The hypothalamus decides how much GnRH to produce based on circulating levels of estrogen and progesterone, as well as numerous other signals, some of which come from the brain. When the pituitary receives GnRH, it looks at other signals coming from the body and produces appropriate amounts of two other important hormones: *follicle-stimulating hormone* (FSH) and *luteinizing hormone* (LH).

Virtually all the systems of your body are affected by the hormones controlled by the hypothalamus and the pituitary gland.

In turn, both FSH and LH signal the ovaries to produce estrogen and progesterone, the hormones responsible for regulating the cyclic changes in the uterus and ovaries. The hypothalamus keeps constant watch over the levels of both estrogen and progesterone, thus creating the mechanism that keeps the hormones in balance throughout the menstrual cycle. As I'll describe in chapter 3, researchers believe that imbalances in these hormones may be responsible for some of the symptoms of PMS. Many of the treatments used for PMS, including the herb black cohosh, affect levels of GnRH, FSH, LH, estrogen, or progesterone.

The hypothalamus plays a key role in regulating the cyclic and hormonal changes that are part of the menstrual cycle.

Calcium is also thought to be an important factor in PMS. Two glands, the thyroid and parathyroid, work together to regulate the amount of calcium in your blood. In chapter 5, we'll talk more about the research showing that supplemental calcium can reduce many PMS symptoms.

The adrenal glands, which lie above the kidneys, also may play a role in PMS through their influence on other hormones. They control a variety of bodily functions by providing hormones to control your blood's mineral content (mineralocorticoids), hormones that affect cell metabolism and your body's response to long-term stress (glucocorticoids), and the sex hormones testosterone and estrogen.

Again, the hypothalamus and pituitary glands monitor the levels of these hormones and substances and help maintain the balance.

The Menstrual Cycle

The purpose of the menstrual cycle is to prepare you for reproduction. From producing an egg and creating the ideal circumstances for fertilization, to readying the uterus to sustain the new life, the menstrual cycle is the key to your reproductive life.

For most women, the menstrual cycle lasts between 25 and 32 days. Although many women focus largely on their periods, menstruation is only a part of the much larger picture. The menstrual cycle actually consists of three distinct and recognizable phases: the follicular phase, ovulation, and the luteal phase.

The Follicular Phase:
The Development of the Ovum

The first day of menstruation marks the beginning of your menstrual cycle. Following the blood loss of menstruation, changes begin in both the ovaries and the lining of the uterus, in preparation for possible pregnancy.

At the beginning of the cycle, the hypothalamus produces GnRH, which signals the pituitary to release FSH. This follicle-stimulating hormone does precisely what its name implies; it stimulates the growth of follicles ("egg containers") in the ovary. This follicle growth is what gives this stage its name. The follicular phase lasts from the first day of your period to ovulation, about 14 days.

Although 10 or 20 follicles may begin to enlarge, usually only one will become dominant and produce an ovum, or egg, ready for fertilization (see figure 2). (If more than one ovum is produced and fertilized, fraternal twins may be the result.) As the follicles develop, they secrete more and more estrogen which, in turn, causes the cells lining the uterus (the endometrium) to multiply, in preparation for possible fertilization. Because

The purpose of the menstrual cycle is to prepare you for reproduction.

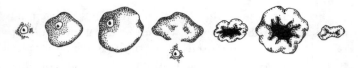

Figure 2. *During the follicular phase, the follicle grows and produces an ovum, which is released during ovulation. Following ovulation, the empty follicle transforms into the corpus luteum.*

this growth of the endometrium is known as *proliferation,* the follicular phase is also known as the proliferative phase.

Ovulation: The Ovum's Release

Ovulation occurs when a follicle ruptures, releasing an ovum. It occurs around the 14th day, right around midcycle.

After its release, the ovum travels along a fallopian tube, reaching the uterus within about 36 hours. Fertilization can take place in the last third of the fallopian tube.

The Luteal Phase: When PMS Can Strike

After ovulation, the menstrual cycle enters what is known as the luteal phase. It is during this phase that you experience PMS. The herb chasteberry (also known as vitex, discussed in chapter 6) is believed to affect hormone levels during this phase of menstruation, thereby reducing symptoms of PMS.

When the follicle ruptures to release the ovum, its outer wall remains behind in the ovary and transforms into a small mass of yellow tissue called the *corpus lu-*

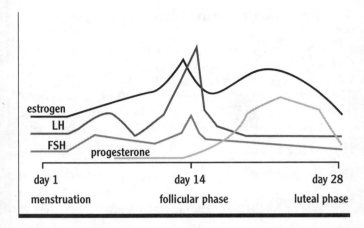

Figure 3. *To prepare your body for possible pregnancy, your glands release hormones that affect the ovaries and the lining of the uterus. The levels of these hormones rise and fall depending on the phase of the cycle.* (Adapted from Nancy Lee Teaf and Kim Wright Wiley, *Perimenopause*, Prima, 1996)

teum. This tissue then begins to secrete the hormone progesterone (see figure 3), which causes glands in the uterine wall to secrete fluid (hence, this is also called the *secretory phase*) and the wall to swell even further.

If fertilization occurs, these changes will allow an egg to become implanted in the endometrium. If pregnancy fails to occur, the secretion of estrogen and progesterone gradually diminishes. No longer needed, the blood-filled uterine lining and the unfertilized egg are shed during menstruation, which occurs about 14 days after the start of ovulation.

With the onset of menstruation and the lowering of estrogen levels, the hypothalamus again signals the pituitary gland to secrete FSH. The cycle begins anew.

Recognizing Your Menstrual Phases

Often, menstruation is the only section of the menstrual cycle we notice. It's not only the most obvious part, but we must do specific things to deal with it. Furthermore, if you

suffer from PMS, your period will no doubt come as a welcome respite from the pain and irritation of PMS. But each phase of your monthly cycle has its own set of clues and effects and, if you take the time to look for them, you'll learn how to recognize all three phases of your menstrual cycle.

If you take the time to look for the clues, you'll learn how to recognize all three phases of your menstrual cycle.

For many women, the follicular phase is notable for its lack of symptoms. For some, the follicular phase actually brings a quiet, deep calm and a sense of well-being. The lightness, energy, confidence, and serenity that you feel during the follicular phase can seem like the polar opposite of PMS.

Ovulation can be easy to notice if you know what to look for. Your ovaries usually take turns releasing an ovum, switching off every month between the right and the left side. Many women notice this happening in their bodies. Some say they feel a very brief "popping" sensation or a cramp coming from one side of the abdomen one month and from the other side the next month. Some notice that this feeling occurs every other month in the same spot.

Even if you do not feel it happening, you can identify ovulation by using the *basal body temperature method*. This involves taking your temperature every morning right when you get up. You will discover that during ovulation, your temperature is about ½ degree Centigrade (1 degree

Fahrenheit) higher than at other times of the month. Your natural lubrication and your saliva will also be clearest and slickest at this time. And often, your sex drive will be strongest around ovulation.

The luteal phase starts right after ovulation. PMS occurs during this time and seems to sneak up on many women. By the time you realize you're experiencing it, you're already knee-deep in PMS, ready to slam the door in irritation at the next person to ring the bell or to crawl back under the bedcovers because all your energy seems to have disappeared. In order to avoid getting yourself into trouble, you might find it helpful to look for the physical clues that may appear after ovulation and before the onset of PMS.

Ovulation can be easy to notice if you know what to look for.

During the luteal phase, your vaginal lubrication is usually thicker and has more of an odor than at other times of the month. Your scalp will also tend to be oilier, and you may notice that your hair seems greasy or flat. Some women find their hair will not hold a perm throughout this time of the month.

One of the most prominent occurrences in the luteal phase is acne, which for some women can occur well into menopause. Because acne may develop even on the scalp, some women purposely wait until after menstruation before coloring their hair.

The PMS Diary

Many of the symptoms of PMS occur in other disorders, so it is vital that you get a sound medical diagnosis. To help your doctor know for sure that you are experiencing PMS and not something else, you might want to keep a "PMS diary."

Angela's Story

Angela's PMS tended to hit her suddenly. She'd be busy at work or at home and suddenly some small annoyance or frustration would send her through the roof. "The rest of the month I can take things in stride," she'd say. "But come PMS time, almost anything can set me off. If my computer locks up at work, I'm ready to smash the screen with a hammer. Once when my daughter disagreed with me about which plates to use to set the table, I found myself screaming at her like she was my enemy. It's terrible." The physical symptoms would soon follow—painful breast tenderness, uncomfortable bloating, and food cravings.

Finally, Angela spoke with her doctor, who suggested that she take calcium. Her doctor told her about a recent study, which found that calcium could improve practically every symptom of PMS, and explained that many of her patients had found it quite helpful. "But it's not perfect," she cautioned Angela. "You really need to keep track of your symptoms, and be prepared to feel emotional a week or so after mid-cycle."

Besides providing your physician with the necessary evidence to diagnose PMS, keeping a PMS diary will mean that *you are now committed to helping yourself feel better.* This single step can provide an important sense of empowerment whereas you once felt only helplessness. Keeping a PMS diary can change your focus from one of passive acceptance to one of action and confrontation.

Later in this chapter, you'll find a sample entry of a PMS diary. To start your own, all you need is a calendar and a notebook or a journal for you to write in daily. Ded-

"How," Angela asked, "am I ever going to know when *that* is?"

It became apparent that Angela had never tracked her menstrual cycle. The doctor explained that while her period was the most noticeable part of her monthly cycle, it was not the only part. She suggested that Angela keep a diary of her monthly symptoms, in an effort to keep track of where she was in her menstrual cycle. "That way you can be prepared. If you know you're about to experience PMS, you can plan on being more emotional, and take that into account."

The calcium helped a lot, but it also helped that Angela became an expert about her own cycle. She could anticipate a time of greater emotional sensitivity and take steps to cope with it. "Now I schedule a massage and a walk with my best friend during the first few days of PMS. I find that if I take care of myself, and also talk about what I'm feeling, everything goes much better." Stories like this are encouraging, but double-blind placebo-controlled studies are the true test of any treatment.

icate a page or so of your notebook or journal to how you feel physically and emotionally each day and note the day's events. Use the calendar to keep track of trends and changes you experience over the long term, as well as mapping out the stages of your menstrual cycle. Once you begin this diary, you may be surprised at the regularity of your pattern of PMS symptoms. You might find it useful to rate the severity of your symptoms. For example, try rating them on a scale from 1 to 3: 1—little bit bothered; 2—bothered; 3—very bothered. This diary will help you recognize the sequence of events of both your menstrual cycle and your PMS.

You are likely to find that your symptoms come in a predictable order. A few days after ovulation, you may no-

You are likely to find that your PMS symptoms come in a pre-dictable order.

tice breast tenderness, followed by constipation. Next, perhaps, you have a headache followed by depression and sporadic bursts of temper. Whatever *your* symptoms, writing them all down is important; include *what* you are experiencing and *when* you are experiencing it.

Once you are sure that you *are* suffering from PMS, you'll be ready to move on to treating this disorder. If you are seeing a physi-

cian, your diary will provide the evidence necessary for him or her to address which treatment may be best for you.

During treatment, it's also important that you continue keeping your PMS diary. This record of PMS-related events will let both you and your physician know how the various treatments are working. Whether your physician prescribes pharmaceuticals or recommends natural products such as calcium supplements, chasteberry, or St. John's wort, your PMS diary will provide the feedback you need to know how successful your therapy has been.

Keeping Your PMS Diary

When you are keeping your PMS diary, noticing not only how you are feeling, but also how the world around is affecting you is important. What you eat, your level of stress, whether you have the flu or a cold—all these things are important and should be a part of your daily diary.

Such events as the seasons of the year, holiday activities, final exams, and important life events (both positive and negative) may also have an effect on your PMS. Stress may play an important role in your PMS, and learning how to best manage it may provide genuine PMS relief. To read about lifestyle changes that can affect PMS, see chapter 11.

Paying attention to how you react to the symptoms of your PMS is also important. Not only do symptoms vary, but not all women react to particular symptoms in the same way. If you become anxious simply *anticipating* the symptoms of PMS before they occur, that reaction particular reaction is worth noting. Once you're aware of such feelings, you can take steps to change or accommodate them. You might also record, for example, your response to increased breast tenderness. Does it cause you

Keeping a careful PMS diary helps you track your symptoms and evaluate whether or not your course of treatment is effective.

discomfort or does it increase your sensuality? (If breast tenderness is one of the more unpleasant of your PMS symptoms, you may find that the herb chasteberry and the supplement evening primrose oil, as well as some of the conventional treatments, may be helpful.)

Your attitude toward your PMS symptoms can also make a big difference in how much the disorder affects you. For example, if you get a PMS headache, does it signal you to slow down and relax before things get out of hand, or does it simply throw you into a funk? Accepting how you feel and stopping to take care of yourself can make a big difference.

Similarly, there is more than one way you can respond to PMS anger. For some women, it can be an exciting, if wholly unsettling, surge of adrenaline. Some women artists even claim to use PMS to enhance their creativity. For most women, however, the anger and extreme emotions are the worst part of PMS and are the symptoms that make them feel so out of control. As we will see in later chapters, several natural treatments may be able to reduce some of the emotional symptoms of PMS.

Your attitude toward your PMS symptoms can make a big difference in how much the disorder affects you.

How you respond to your symptoms will become apparent in your diary. Avoid being judgmental about what you're experiencing. Don't view your reactions as either good or bad. Remember that your emotions and actions are the result of a complex mix of causes and that they are related to the physical disorder of PMS.

You might wish to involve your partner or family members in helping you keep track of your PMS. Sometimes, others who spend time with us are able to see things that we find simply "too close" to notice. Those around you may also be better able to notice whether or not a particular treatment may be relieving some of your symptoms. For example, if you try St. John's wort for your PMS depression, someone in your family may be first to notice improvement. However, be careful and be clear in requesting help with your diary. Remind those you live with that you are looking for observations, not for interpretations or judgments.

Finally, think of your PMS diary as a long-term friend, one in whom you can confide. You may, like some women, find your PMS diary so helpful that you'll want to keep one for the rest of your reproductive years. Here are some suggestions to help you get started.

- Keep track of what is happening to you throughout the monthly cycle; include both emotional and physical symptoms, periods of stress, seasonal activities, illness, and important life changes.
- Write down your own reactions to your symptoms of PMS.
- Note what treatments you use to relieve your symptoms (herbs, exercise, dietary changes, supplements, stress reduction) and your reactions to them.
- Avoid being judgmental about what you are experiencing and how you react to your experiences.
- Use your partner or family to help you keep track of your symptoms, your reactions to them, and, with treatment, any improvement they might notice.

The Diary
Here's a sample entry from a PMS diary. You may find it useful in setting up your own PMS diary.

June 16
Symptoms
Felt tired today and became angry very easily (worth about a 2 rating). Had a headache during the morning, but it left by lunch. Experienced a wild craving for chocolate chips (definitely rated a 3!).

Reactions
Felt a bit guilty for snapping at the kids this morning. They weren't out of control, just noisy. I apologized later and read them a story. That headache just seemed to drain my strength and my patience, and I never really regained my usual energy. If I had had the oomph, I would have

gone to the store to get those chips, but (luckily, I guess) I never made it.

Meals/Snacks

Breakfast: Coffee, orange, toast with margarine, half a container of blueberry yogurt

Snack: Carrots and apple juice

Lunch: Half a turkey sandwich with mayonnaise and mustard; small salad with lowfat dressing

Dinner: Burrito Night! (made with tortillas, refried beans, Cheddar cheese, tomatoes, olives), milk; applesauce with cinnamon for dessert

Treatments

Tried Advil for headache (it finally kicked in about 11:30 A.M.).

Put the twins down for a nap and managed a half hour of yoga—it seemed to help, I wasn't as tense as I was this morning.

Sources of Stress

Babysitter cancelled for tomorrow night. Called three replacements with no luck until Mom agreed to watch the kids. Had long discussion with Mom about whose house would host Nora's birthday party—enough said! Dry cleaner lost two buttons on my dress for Bob's client dinner tomorrow. Couldn't find the utilities bill until after the postman picked up the mail. Dog got loose and I had to chase him down.

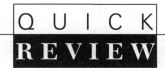

QUICK REVIEW

- Understanding your menstrual cycle is an important first step in learning to treat your PMS.
- The menstrual cycle is a monthly process governed by a complex interaction of hormones, involving estrogen and progesterone, under the control of the hypothalamus and pituitary gland.
- The menstrual cycle has three distinct phases: the follicular phase, ovulation, and the luteal phase. PMS and its symptoms occur *only* during the luteal phase, which takes place during the 14 days prior to menstruation.
- Each of the menstrual cycle's three phases presents its own unique signs and clues. By paying close attention and knowing what to look for, you can learn to recognize each phase.
- Keeping a PMS diary is an excellent way to begin taking control of your PMS. It will help you and your physician diagnose as well as treat your symptoms and, following treatment, enable you to evaluate how effective each therapy is.

What Causes PMS?

olly's job evaluation did not go well. Her boss said that her headaches and absences detracted from her job performance. What's more, he continued, her mood swings and crying spells disrupted the entire office staff. When she mentioned that these problems were due to her PMS, he gave her a skeptical, it's-all-in-your-head look.

Molly was beside herself. She felt as though the world was against her, that her PMS was ruining her life, and that no one seemed to care.

Few people would tell a woman with asthma that her wheezing was just a ploy to get attention, or ask a man with prostate disease to stop using the restroom so frequently. But perhaps because PMS has no known cause and because it involves emotions, other people often believe a woman experiencing PMS should somehow be able to snap out of it. Whatever their reasons, our coworkers, family members, sometimes even our women friends are often insensitive about PMS.

If you are like Molly, knowing that premenstrual syndrome is a real physical disorder with symptoms that can be treated, even though we don't understand what causes them, is important. Not knowing the exact cause of a disorder doesn't necessarily prevent us from finding effective treatments for it. Consider high blood pressure, for example. In the overwhelming majority of cases, the reason for a person's high blood pressure cannot be identified. Yet dozens of effective drugs can lower elevated blood pressure.

While we may not understand the origin of PMS or precisely why some of the treatments work, what is important is that they *do* work.

So it is with premenstrual syndrome. We may not understand its origin and may not know why some herbs or medications can help the symptoms, but what matters is that the treatments *do* work—that there *is* relief for your PMS. Also, because some treatments work so well for certain symptoms of PMS, they can tell us important things about this disorder and what may cause it.

Major Theories About the Causes of PMS

Medical researchers have suggested several possible causes of PMS. The major theories are as follows:

- Calcium deficiency
- Estrogen imbalance
- Overproduction of prolactin
- Abnormal levels of essential fatty acids
- Decreased progesterone

To Treat an Illness, One Need Not Know Its Cause

We do not have to know the cause of PMS to treat the condition. Many disorders for which the causes are not known can nonetheless be treated effectively. Depression is a good example. While we have many ideas about what may cause depression, we have no definitive explanation.

Still, antidepressants such as Prozac and Zoloft are known to provide help for those suffering from severe depression. One herbal product, St. John's wort, has been found to help those suffering from mild to moderate depression. What's remarkable is that even though we aren't sure exactly how these treatments act on depression, there's plenty of evidence that they help.

Calcium Deficiency: Affects More Than Just Your Bones

Due to the results of one important study, a previously minor theory about the cause of PMS has suddenly taken center stage. For years, a few researchers have believed that calcium played a major role in PMS, but the idea was not well known outside of this small circle of scientists. This changed with the publication of a large and well-designed study in 1998. This groundbreaking work found that calcium supplements can reduce almost all the symptoms of PMS.[1]

We don't really know why calcium is so important in PMS, but we have several clues that link the two. One is the similarity between PMS symptoms and the signs of severe calcium deficiency, which include agitation, irritability, and depression.[2,3]

Furthermore, low levels of calcium are known to occur during PMS. These low levels in turn stimulate an overproduction of parathyroid hormone, one of the major calcium-regulating hormones. Increased levels of parathyroid hormone are known to affect mood and mental function, perhaps through an interaction with serotonin.[4,5]

Additional evidence for a PMS-calcium connection is suggested by studies that show a relationship between PMS symptoms and the later development of osteoporosis.[6,7] In fact, it may be that PMS symptoms are actually an early sign of calcium deficiency.

It may be that PMS symptoms are actually an early sign of calcium deficiency.

We'll talk more about calcium and its effect on PMS, and how you can use this safe and healthful supplement to treat your PMS symptoms, in chapter 5.

Estrogen Imbalance: Too Much Estrogen, Too Little Progesterone

Researchers have long thought that the hormone estrogen may be the key to premenstrual syndrome. One of the leading theories about PMS is based on the fact that during the last 2 weeks of the menstrual cycle (the time during which you experience PMS), some women with PMS have an overabundance of estrogen *in relation* to the amount of progesterone.[8] One treatment based on this concept is the use of oral contraceptives. However, in practice, it produces mixed results.

"The pill" contains both estrogen and progesterone, thereby altering the natural ratio of these hormones. Experience has shown that using oral contraceptives can

Debunking the Myths About PMS

Susan just didn't *believe* in PMS. "Come on now," she would say to her women colleagues, "don't you agree that PMS is just a cover for female neurosis?" She was completely serious. Unlike millions of other women, she had never experienced PMS.

Susan's attitude toward PMS is not unusual. Until only a few decades ago, PMS was referred to as "female hysteria" or "melancholia." Physicians didn't believe that it was even a medical condition at all. Women were simply considered "too emotional."

Today, however, we know that PMS is real and that it affects millions of women. But the history of ignorance about PMS lives on. Here are some of the modern myths about PMS.

It's All in Your Head

It's not unusual for friends and family to mistake the symptoms of PMS for the results of unresolved emotional or psychological trauma. In effect, they think there is something

dramatically help some women with their symptoms of PMS, but this treatment fails completely for others, sometimes even making symptoms worse. The reason for this could be that oral contraceptive therapy doesn't really *balance* the hormones, as some suggest, but merely *changes* them around. The change is apparently helpful only for some women.

Properly analyzing how estrogen affects a woman's body is difficult because the changes it brings about are so far-reaching. Besides playing an important role in the wrong with you mentally. Obviously such people do not understand the physical nature of PMS. While science is not sure of its exact cause, PMS is, without doubt, a physical condition. Like asthma or Parkinson's disease, PMS has a complex biological origin. Just as you would not consider telling someone with Parkinson's that his disorder was purely psychological, the same should be true for PMS.

If You Manage Your Life Better, You Wouldn't Have PMS

Some people seem to believe that if a woman could just be more efficient, she wouldn't be overwhelmed by the mood swings or feel the fatigue that we now recognize as PMS symptoms. However, the opposite is more often true: When you get PMS, managing your life can become impossible. We know that PMS is not the result of a lack of organization; rather, it is the outcome of a complex scenario of hormonal interactions that take place in the brain.

(continued)

menstrual cycle, estrogen maintains the tissues of your reproductive system—the walls that line the vagina and the uterus, and the cells of the inside of the fallopian tubes. Estrogen in the kidneys can cause sodium and water retention, leading to swelling in the hands and feet. This hormone also protects blood vessels from atherosclerosis (hardening of the arteries) and preserves the bones from osteoporosis. But on the other hand, estrogen contributes to the growth of hormone-sensitive cancers in the breast and uterus.

Debunking the Myths About PMS *(continued)*
If You Diet, You Won't Gain Water Weight

Diet is not the primary cause of excessive water-weight gain during PMS. Instead, the pounds you might gain during PMS are most likely the result of internal hormonal messages. However, your weight can also be affected if you eat a lot of salt. If weight gain during PMS is a problem for you, learn which foods to avoid. You might also consider trying ginkgo, which appears to be helpful for many symptoms of fluid retention.

Estrogen can also affect neurotransmitters such as serotonin, chemicals that play an important role in mood and mental function.[9,10] This may explain why antidepressant drugs such as Prozac and Zoloft are helpful in PMS; they, too, affect serotonin. So does the herb St. John's wort. To read more about St. John's wort and how it may be useful in PMS depression, see chapter 10.

Overproduction of Prolactin: A Cause of Breast Tenderness?

Prolactin is the hormone that stimulates milk production and the other breast changes necessary to prepare for breastfeeding. Excessive production of prolactin (a condition known as *hyperprolactinemia*) can cause breast swelling and tenderness, as well as other PMS symptoms.[11]

The herb chasteberry, also known as vitex, reduces prolactin levels,[12] and is a widely used treatment in Germany for cyclic breast tenderness and other PMS symptoms. To learn more about chasteberry and its use in treating PMS, see chapter 6. Conventional drugs that re-

You're Just Using PMS As an Excuse

Some people react to your PMS in this way: "You're just using PMS as an excuse to unload your bad mood on me." They seem to believe that women use PMS as an excuse for emotional outbursts, so that we can claim the "PMS defense" when we feel upset. However, they overlook one crucial point: We don't act this way by choice! This attitude reflects these people's inability to cope with the simple realities of someone else's illness.

duce prolactin levels, such as bromocriptine, also seem to be effective in treating some symptoms of PMS. However, as with all the other theories about PMS, we have many gaps in our knowledge about the relationship between PMS symptoms and prolactin.

Essential Fatty Acids: Known to Affect Inflammation and Pain

Even though we are told that fats are bad for us, this is not the case for all of them. *Essential fatty acids* (or EFAs) are important fats that we require in order to stay healthy. Because our bodies are not able to synthesize them, we must obtain essential fatty acids from our diet. EFAs play a number of roles in the body, but the one relevant to PMS concerns the effects of EFAs on substances known as *prostaglandins* and *leukotrienes*. These are natural substances that influence inflammation and pain. Some of them decrease inflammation while others increase it. Women with PMS may have an imbalance in EFAs, leading to increased inflammation in the breast as well as other symptoms of PMS.[13]

Evening primrose oil is a good source of the major EFA gamma-linolenic acid (GLA). Long-term use of evening primrose oil may tend to help PMS symptoms (especially breast discomfort) by normalizing EFA levels.[14] For more information about treating PMS with evening primrose oil, see chapter 7.

Low Progesterone: A Cause of Anxiety?

Some researchers believe that low levels of progesterone may be indirectly responsible for some of the emotional symptoms of PMS. When progesterone levels drop, so do levels of a related hormone called allopregnanolone. Researchers think that reduced allopregnanolone levels may cause anxiety or depression, because allopregnanolone appears to have an effect on an important neurotransmitter known as GABA (gamma-aminobutyric acid).[15,16]

Long-term use of evening primrose oil may help PMS symptoms (especially breast discomfort) by normalizing EFA levels.

GABA plays a role in anxiety at least as important as serotonin's role in depression (most drugs used to treat anxiety work by enhancing the action of GABA). When allopregnanolone levels fall, GABA may be adversely affected, bringing about symptoms of anxiety.

However, while progesterone, the source of allopregnanolone, has long been used as a treatment for PMS symptoms, it doesn't appear to be very effective.[17]

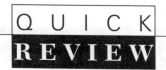

QUICK
REVIEW

- Although we may not understand the cause of PMS, treatments that can be effective in relieving many of its symptoms are available.

- The major theories about the causes of PMS include calcium deficiency, estrogen imbalance, overproduction of prolactin, abnormal levels of essential fatty acids, and decreased progesterone.

- Recent evidence suggests that calcium may also play a major role in PMS. According to a major new study, calcium supplementation can significantly reduce the symptoms of PMS.

- A leading theory about the cause of PMS is that, during the last 2 weeks of your monthly cycle (during which you experience PMS), estrogen is overabundant in relation to progesterone.

- Serotonin levels may be involved in PMS depression. Antidepressant drugs in the Prozac family, as well as the herb St. John's wort, affect serotonin levels, and may be helpful for PMS depression.

- The hormone prolactin may also play a role in PMS symptoms, especially breast tenderness. The herb chasteberry works by affecting prolactin levels.

- Because essential fatty acids (EFAs) are out of balance in women with PMS, supplementation with evening primrose oil (a good source of EFAs) appears to reduce cyclic breast tenderness (for more information, see the discussion in chapter 7).

- Some researchers believe that low levels of progesterone may cause some of the depression and anxiety of PMS. Progesterone supplementation does not, however, appear to be an effective treatment for PMS.

Conventional
Treatment for PMS

C onventional medicine has a difficult time treating
PMS. While this is in part because we don't fully
understand the precise cause of PMS, it's also because PMS involves such a variety of symptoms. As yet,
we have no "magic potion" for curing PMS, although, as
we'll see in chapter 5, the supplement calcium is looking
awfully promising.

Your doctor's approach will be to treat specific symptoms, most likely the ones that are bothering you most.
For the emotional ups and downs of PMS, he might prescribe one of the new generation of antidepressants such
as Prozac or Zoloft. For bloating and water-weight gain,
your doctor may suggest a diuretic (water pill) such as
Lasix. If these medications either fail to help you or actually make things worse, your doctor may suggest other
pharmaceuticals, including hormone therapies. Some of
these drugs may be used in combinations. Although these
drugs may relieve your symptoms, their side effects can

also cause problems of their own, adding to your usual assortment of PMS difficulties.

That PMS is so difficult to treat has also made physicians more willing to experiment with new and unconventional therapies. While your doctor may recommend antidepressants, pain relievers, or hormones, he or she also may guide you toward calcium supplements, vitamins, evening primrose oil, or other natural products. If not, you may wish to inquire about them specifically, perhaps mentioning the natural treatments discussed in this book.

Although modern medicine can treat the symptoms of PMS, there is no "magic potion" to cure the condition.

Your initial visit to your doctor is the starting point of discovering which medications will work best for you. Your physician will draw upon a large and varied "medicine chest" of possibilities. The variety of pharmaceutical treatments commonly used for PMS include the following:

- Antidepressants
- Hormone therapies
- Antianxiety drugs
- Diuretics
- Headache medication

This chapter, then, will cover the *conventional* medical treatments for PMS, including how each drug can help you, what side effects you may experience, and, in general, what the modern pharmacopoeia has to offer to treat the many and varied symptoms of PMS. In subsequent chapters, I'll discuss alternatives to these treatments—the numerous safe and natural herbal products and dietary supplements that can be of great benefit in treating your premenstrual syndrome. For all treatments, whether pharmaceutical or natural, I'll explain how each works and tell you about the scientific research that supports its use. I'll also discuss the nature of scientific research itself.

Antidepressants

Depression is one of the most common complaints of PMS. Linda, a housewife and mother of four, is a good example of this. Linda is almost always able to handle the day-to-day demands of a busy household: preparing meals, shopping, and driving the kids back and forth from school, soccer games, and gymnastics lessons. During a week or two each month, however, things are different.

"I wish I could just be alone when I get PMS," she says. "I just want to hide and not have to face anyone."

The intensity of Linda's PMS varies from month to month. At its best, Linda's PMS depression leaves her feeling listless and gloomy. Sometimes she feels continually fatigued. The demands of her family seem almost too much to bear. At its worst, Linda becomes overly emotional: sad, tearful, crying for no apparent reason, and on the verge of being completely overwhelmed by hopelessness.

Depression is surprisingly common. One out of every six persons experiences an episode of serious depression at some time during their lives, and many more experience periods of mild to moderate depression. PMS depression, however, is different in that it occurs *only during one particular time of the monthly cycle:* from 1 to 14 days prior to your period.

If you feel depressed at other times of the month (or throughout the month), it is very unlikely that your depression is caused by PMS. I recommend you seek professional help, as there are many effective treatments for depression. (For more information on both conventional and natural options for depression, see *The Natural Pharmacist Guide to St. John's Wort and Depression.*)

Tricyclics and SSRIs: Enter Prozac

PMS depression, however, is different in that it occurs only during one particular time of the monthly cycle: from 1 to 14 days prior to menstruation.

Prior to the mid-1980s, the main type of antidepressant medication in use was a class of drugs called the *tricyclics.* These medications raise brain levels of several chemicals, such as serotonin, norepinephrine, and dopamine. Some commonly known tricyclic antidepressants include Elavil, Sinequan, and Tofranil.

Although tricyclics have been successful in treating serious depression, they can cause numerous side effects including fatigue, drowsiness, blurred vision, weight gain, dizziness, and heart palpitations.

One of the reasons tricyclic drugs cause so many side effects is that they work in shotgun-like manner: They affect so many chemicals at once that undesired consequences are inevitable. In the mid-1980s, a new type of antidepressant came on the scene—one that focused quite specifically on only one brain chemical, serotonin. These *selective serotonin-reuptake inhibitors* (named after the way they affect serotonin) cause far fewer side effects than the tricyclics. It is this family of antidepressants that is being used most often to treat the depression associated with PMS.[1]

The well-known drug Prozac (fluoxetine) is a member of this category of antidepressants. After it became available, Prozac was so widely used for depression that it gained something of a celebrity status. Other SSRIs include the drugs Zoloft (sertraline hydrochloride) and Paxil (paroxetine).

Can Antidepressants Help PMS?

Antidepressant drugs have provided enormous benefits to millions of depressed people. But can they help with the kind of short-term depression caused by PMS, which lasts from only a few days to a few weeks? The answer appears to be yes. Good scientific evidence indicates that certain antidepressants can provide relief for some of the depression-like symptoms of PMS.

Numerous studies tell us that Prozac can reduce the anxiety, depression, and irritability that are part of PMS.[2-8] Other studies have shown that Prozac, Zoloft, and Paxil can help PDD as well, a form of PMS with more severe symptoms.[9-12] (See chapter 1 for more information on PDD.)

Although tricyclics treat serious depression, they can cause numerous side effects.

Antidepressant drugs are slow acting. Unlike taking aspirin, which will relieve headaches within an hour or so, you may have to take these medications daily for 4 to 6 weeks before you experience relief. Using antidepressants this way may make perfect sense for ordinary chronic depression, which tends to last for months, but for PMS it presents a problem. PMS depression occurs only for a week or two each month. Since these drugs usually take so long to work, you may have to take them day in and day out throughout the month to treat 1 week of depression. This is a big drawback, because most people don't like to take medications every day when they don't feel sick.

However, more recent studies suggest that these drugs might work more quickly for PMS depression than for other forms of depression.[13] In a 1994 study, a group of women with PDD were given Prozac only during the last 2 weeks of their periods, the luteal phase when PMS symptoms occur. More than half the women experienced complete relief and almost one-third experienced partial but significant relief. A second study arrived at similar conclusions.[14] It may be that for PMS depression you can get away with taking medications on more of an "as needed" basis.

Many women who take Prozac can't achieve orgasm while on the medication.

However, these studies have met with some skepticism from physicians. More research needs to be done to clarify the issue.

The Side Effects of SSRIs

Although Prozac and the other SSRIs were a big advance over previous medications, they still cause side effects. If your doctor chooses to treat your PMS depression with one of these drugs, you will have to decide whether the possible improvement outweighs the side effects that may result.

The most intrusive side effect is sexual dysfunction. An estimated 30% of women who take Prozac and other SSRIs can't achieve orgasm while they are on the medication.[15] This is one of the most common reasons that women stop taking such drugs.

Insomnia is another common side effect of SSRIs, as are headaches, drowsiness, nausea, and an uncomfortable, agitated feeling. Many of these side effects, however, may disappear after a few weeks. If they do not disappear, switching to a different SSRI may—or may not—solve the problem.

Another option might be switching to St. John's wort. Strong scientific evidence tells us that this virtually side-effect–free herb is an effective treatment for mild to moderate depression. While it hasn't been tested specifically for PMS depression, it is logical to assume that it should help. For more information on St. John's wort and depression, see chapter 10.

Oral contraceptives affect PMS by reducing the levels of hormones related to ovulation, which can sometimes reduce symptoms.

Hormone Therapies

Since PMS is clearly related to women's hormones, the most obvious way to treat PMS is to use therapies that affect hormones. However, these treatments have far-reaching consequences, which is why many physicians try antidepressant therapy first (as you will see in chapter 5, calcium may be even a better option). Oral contraceptive pills are often the next choice.

The Pill: Provides Relief for Some Women

Oral contraceptives contain enough estrogen and progesterone to dramatically change the hormonal landscape of your body. The net effect is to reduce levels of FSH and LH, two natural hormones related to ovulation. Although periods don't stop, PMS symptoms sometimes decrease.

A 1992 double-blind placebo-controlled trial following 82 women found that certain oral contraceptives reduce

Marsha's Story

When Marsha was younger, she'd watched her older sister Jennifer go through the difficult process of trying to control her PMS. Valium made Jennifer dopey, the pill made her symptoms worse, and Prozac. . . . "Well," Jennifer had told young Marsha, "when you get older you'll understand why I didn't like Prozac." What she didn't want to mention was that Prozac made her unable to experience an orgasm.

You can probably understand why Marsha was so nervous when, years later, she visited her doctor in search of solutions for her PMS. She was afraid that if the symptoms kept up, she wouldn't have any friends left. "I scream like a raving maniac," she admitted. "Everything makes me blow up. And I'm so bloated I feel like I'm going to pop."

Her doctor was understanding. He told her that with a disorder like PMS, she'd need a solution that would be both safe and effective for many years.

PMS symptoms, particularly breast pain and weight gain.[16] Another study of 37 women also found benefits.[17]

Birth control pills do appear to alleviate some of the symptoms of PMS in some women. However, birth control pills don't specifically balance hormones. Rather, they simply change them around. For this reason, some women feel no noticeable effect, while others report that their symptoms of PMS become even worse.

Oral contraceptives can also cause various side effects, including nausea, weight gain, depression, cramps, headaches, dizziness, blood clots, and breast swelling.

"I've read a recent study that suggests calcium supplements can help with a lot of the problems you're having with PMS," he told her. "More than half of the women taking calcium in this study reported real improvement in their symptoms of PMS. The great thing about taking calcium is that it's safe and virtually free of side effects. And what's more, taking it will help you keep up your calcium levels as you get older and face the risk of osteoporosis."

Marsha took 1,200 mg a day of calcium in the form of calcium carbonate. Although she noticed no benefit at first, by the end of two menstrual cycles, her symptoms had been dramatically reduced.

"It's like the difference between night and day," she says. "I still get a little grumpy around my period, but my symptoms are nothing compared to what they were before."

We'll review the evidence for calcium in the next chapter. As we shall see, a major research study suggests that calcium supplements may be the most important treatment to try for PMS.

What About Progesterone Alone?

For decades, some physicians have prescribed progesterone alone (or hormones related to it, known as progestins) for the treatment of PMS. However, evidence suggests that this approach is not any better than placebo treatment.[18,19]

Danocrine: Actually Stops Menstruation

Another hormone therapy is Danocrine (danazol). Danocrine is a synthetic hormone related to testosterone, the so-called male sex hormone that is actually produced naturally in both men and women. Danocrine also reduces the levels of FSH and LH sufficiently to cause the menstrual period to actually stop. The net effect is simple—no periods, no PMS. A 1990 trial reported that when 21 women with PMS were given Danocrine, PMS symptoms were reduced by as much as 85%.[20] Good results were also seen in another small study.[21]

Side effects of Danocrine include dizziness, changes in appetite, anxiety, fluid retention, sexual dysfunction, and changes in sleep patterns. About 80% of women taking danazol experience weight gain or acne. Danocrine can also cause the growth of body hair in women and may even deepen the voice. Symptoms of menopause, such as vaginal dryness and hot flashes may also occur. However, these symptoms will disappear when Danocrine therapy is stopped.

Pregnant women cannot use danazol since it can "masculinize" a female fetus. Danocrine can also affect an infant through breast milk.

Although Danocrine effectively relieves PMS symptoms by halting menstruation, not all women wish to resort to such extreme measures. If you'd like to consider some alternatives to the hormone therapies I've just described, some of the natural treatments described in later chapters might be of aid. For example, black cohosh is believed to block the effect of estrogen while exerting some estrogen-like effects itself. Chasteberry (vitex) works in a completely different way: It reduces levels of the hormone prolactin. The big advantage of these two treatments is that they appear to be nearly side-effect free. For more information about them, see chapter 6 for chasteberry, and chapter 9 for black cohosh.

Antianxiety Medications

Nervousness and anxiety are two common complaints about PMS. As I mentioned in chapter 1, these symptoms range from feelings of irritability and worry to panic attacks. Some of the conventional treatments for PMS-related anxiety include benzodiazepines, BuSpar, and beta-blockers. These medications provide fairly prompt relief, although only the benzodiazepine Xanax has been specifically tested in PMS. However, BuSpar and beta-blockers are also believed to be effective. Similarly, a natural treatment widely prescribed in Europe for anxiety, kava, is reportedly effective even though it too has not been tested for use in PMS.

Xanax, one of the most common benzodiazepines, may significantly reduce PMS anxiety.

Benzodiazepines: May Help Anxiety, but Can Be Addictive

Anxiety in PMS is treated largely with one particular family of sedatives called *benzodiazepines.* Although you may not have heard of this group of drugs, you probably are familiar with its best known member, Valium (diazepam). Other commonly used benzodiazepines include Xanax (alprazolam), Librium (chlordiazepoxide hydrochloride), and Ativan (lorazepam). Because the use of these drugs carries some risk of addiction, there is considerable controversy regarding their use in treating the relatively mild symptoms of PMS.

Xanax is one of the most commonly prescribed benzodiazepines for PMS anxiety. Two double-blind studies have demonstrated that 0.25 mg of Xanax 4 times a day, used only during the last 2 weeks of the menstrual cycle, significantly reduces PMS anxiety.[22]

Benzodiazepine drugs are sedatives. However, they don't put you to sleep. Xanax is actually a very subtle drug. Side

effects include light-headedness, dizziness, depression, confusion, clumsiness, and fatigue. Alcohol, barbiturates, and
antihistamines can all increase the effects of these drugs.

BuSpar: Slow-Acting, but Effective Relief

BuSpar (buspirone) is a nonbenzodiazepine drug that can
also help anxiety. Although we don't really know how it

works, BuSpar is a uniquely non-
addictive and non-sedating antianxiety treatment. BuSpar has
not been specifically tested in
PMS, but many physicians believe that it is effective.

> **Inderal is report-
> edly helpful for
> PMS, although
> there has been
> little specific scien-
> tific investigation
> of its effectiveness.**

One of the big advantages
with BuSpar is that it seldom
causes severe side effects. However, a few people feel tired,
dizzy, headachy, or nauseous
when they take it. BuSpar's only
downside is that it is somewhat
slow acting, requiring at least
one week to reach its full effect.

Beta-Blockers: Not Just for Hypertension

Inderal (propranolol) is another nonbenzodiazepine that
is sometimes used for treating anxiety. Originally developed for the treatment of hypertension and angina, Inderal and related drugs (known as *beta-blockers*) slow the
heart rate and suppress other physical symptoms of anxiety. Reportedly, these drugs are helpful for PMS, although
there has been little specific scientific investigation of
their effectiveness.

Beta-blockers can cause fatigue, weakness, depression,
asthma, excessively slow heart rate, and gastrointestinal
distress.

Diuretics

Fluid retention is another common complaint of PMS. During the luteal phase of their cycle, women often feel bloated and uncomfortably distended. Diuretic drugs are sometimes prescribed to women who suffer from this symptom. The action of diuretic drugs is quite simple: They increase the amount of fluid that is urinated.

Lasix (furosemide), Aldactone (spironolactone), and metolazone are the most commonly prescribed diuretics for PMS. A Swedish study of 35 women found that Aldactone, when taken only during the period of PMS bloating, relieved not only PMS, but also emotional symptoms, breast tenderness, and food cravings.[23] Why a diuretic should help other symptoms besides fluid retention is a mystery.

Diuretics can cause loss of potassium, which can be dangerous. Natural treatments that may be able to reduce the fluid retention associated with PMS without causing any significant side effects include calcium and ginkgo. See chapters 5 and 9 for more information on these options.

Headache Medication

Imitrex (sumatriptan) is a medicine well known for its use in migraine headaches. It is often used to treat premenstrual headaches as well. In one study, sumatriptan was used to treat premenstrual migraines that were not responding to over-the-counter medications such as aspirin or Aleve (naproxen sodium). When used by 42 women with PMS over a period of 12 months, sumatriptan relieved headaches 80% of the time. Less than half of the participants reported mild side effects, such as tightness around the head and neck, fatigue, and nausea.[24]

In addition, drugs that can help prevent migraine headaches can be helpful for women who suffer from PMS. Inderal, Prozac, and ergot drugs such as ergotamine are among the most commonly used.

The supplement magnesium and the herb feverfew can also be used to prevent migraine headaches, as will be described in chapters 8 and 10.

Desperate Measures

In some cases, PMS can be so severe that women are willing to do almost anything to make its symptoms go away. If the therapies previously described in this chapter fail to work, and if a woman is truly desperate, a doctor may recommend surgical removal of her ovaries.

The drugs Buserelin and Leuprolide, also called GnRH inhibitors, can provide a less final but still drastic solution. By entirely shutting off FSH and LH, these drugs essentially put women into early menopause. (For more information on menopause, see *The Natural Pharmacist Guide to Menopause.*)

A Word About Research

As you've probably already noticed, throughout this book I will be using terms such as "anecdotal evidence," "placebo effect," and "double-blind placebo-controlled study," to discuss the evidence for and against treatments for PMS. I'd like to take the time to describe why such research is important and what these terms mean.

Anecdotal Evidence

For generations, our ancestors have relied on word-of-mouth recommendations for much of their health care. The official name for this type of information is *anecdotal evidence.* For example, Aunt June tells you that feverfew has cured her migraine headaches, or your brother Bob describes the miraculous results he got by taking glucosamine and chondroitin for his painful shoulder. Although definitely not solid scientific evidence, anecdotes can be quite valuable. In many cases, it is through such practical experience that we first discover the treatments that are worth investigating.

However, through hard experience, scientists have discovered many flaws in this word-of-mouth system. When Aunt June reported that feverfew worked for her, how can we know for certain whether it was actually the herb that made the difference? Maybe it was because she moved to Florida at the same time. Or was her life less stressful than usual? There are many factors to consider.

The Placebo Effect

Scientists discovered long ago that even ineffective treatments can produce dramatic benefits in many people. We know this from studies where people are given placebo pills—fake treatments disguised as real ones. This is known as the _placebo effect,_ and most people find it hard to accept just how powerful it can be. Depending on the condition, as many as 30 to 70% of people participating in a study may report great results with a phony pill![25,26] Furthermore, contrary to popular belief, the placebo effect does not necessarily wear off in time. According to some studies, placebo pills can continue to produce benefits for years, as long as you _believe_ that you are taking real medicine.

This factor can make anecdotes very misleading. If 100 people are given placebos, 30 to 70 of them will be able to give enthusiastic testimonials!

Double-Blind Placebo-Controlled Study

Because of the confusion caused by the placebo effect, researchers gradually developed a standard system to truly find out whether a treatment is working based on its own powers. This method is called a *double-blind placebo-controlled study.* In such a trial, the participants are given either real treatment or phony treatment (the placebo control), and neither the study's participants nor the researchers know which is which (both participants and researchers are "blind").

Keeping both doctors and participants in the dark is essential. If participants knew they were receiving a

Safety is as important as effectiveness when using any kind of medication or treatment.

placebo, it wouldn't make them feel better. Likewise, if researchers knew who was getting the real treatment, they might inadvertently give subtle hints that would tip off the participants, or they might unconsciously bias their evaluation of participant recovery.

A double-blind study lets researchers separate the placebo effect from the real value of a treatment. When two groups of people take pills that they all know *might or might not* be a treatment, and the group receiving real treatment does much better than the other, we can begin to feel confident that the treatment might be helpful in itself.

When a study involves enough participants (a minimum of 100 is usually suggested), it can allow us to arrive at conclusions that are quite reliable. Nonetheless, scientific research can't predict how well a treatment will work for *you.* Everyone is unique. Even with the best of studies, doctors must frequently rely on the process of trial and error.

What About Safety?

When it comes to medication, safety is as important as effectiveness. Whether you are using a prescribed medication, an over-the-counter drug, or an herbal product, finding something that actually *works* is important. But it is just as vital that the treatment you use be a safe one.

Almost all medications have side effects, some of which can be serious. Natural products are no exception. Before you take any medication, you should evaluate the benefits against the possible risks. Issues to consider include annoying side effects, serious risks, possibility of overdose, interactions with medications you may already be taking, and long-term safety. It is also important to know that no matter how safe a medication can be in general, the risk that a single individual might have an unusually bad reaction to it is always there.

The FDA makes sure that all known safety issues regarding drugs are available to pharmacists, doctors, and the public. It is much more difficult to obtain information on the safety of herbs and natural supplements. In the remaining chapters of this book, I will explain what is known about the risks and side effects of these natural treatments.

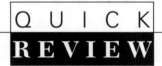

■ The antidepressant Prozac and other drugs in the SSRI family have been shown to be effective in treating PMS depression. Ordinarily, such medications must be taken continuously for a period of at least 4 to 6 weeks to provide benefits. However, interesting new evidence suggests that you may be able to take these medications just during the period of PMS instead.

- The main problem with SSRI antidepressants is that they can cause up to 30% of women taking them to be unable to achieve orgasm. Other possible side effects are headaches, nausea, drowsiness, insomnia, and an uncomfortable, agitated feeling.

- Birth control pills do appear to alleviate some of the symptoms of PMS in some women.

- Danocrine halts menstruation, and likewise PMS, but can cause dizziness, changes in appetite, anxiety, fluid retention, sexual dysfunction, changes in sleep patterns, weight gain, acne, vaginal dryness, hot flashes, growth of body hair, and deepening of voice in some women. Pregnant women should not take Danocrine because it can masculinize a female fetus.

- Antianxiety medications, such as benzodiazepines, BuSpar, and beta-blockers, can also be helpful. One of the most commonly used benzodiazepine is Xanax. Some people taking benzodiazepines may experience light-headedness, dizziness, depression, confusion, clumsiness, and fatigue. Such medications can be addictive and may interact with alcohol, barbiturates, and antihistamines. Beta-blockers can cause fatigue, weakness, depression, asthma, excessively slow heart rate, and gastrointestinal distress. BuSpar is relative safe but is slow acting.

- Diuretics such as Lasix (furosemide) and Aldactone (spironolactone) may be helpful for women for whom fluid retention is the predominant symptom of PMS. Diuretics can cause potassium loss, which could be dangerous.

- Headache medications, most notably the common migraine drug sumatriptan, can offer effective treatment for PMS headaches.

- Severe PMS may require drastic measures such as removal of ovaries or use of drugs that result in early menopause.
- Natural treatments that appear to provide many of these same benefits without significant side effects are described in the next chapters.

Calcium

The PMS Breakthrough

Women have long been encouraged to supplement their diets with calcium in order to prevent osteoporosis. Until recently, however, calcium was seldom mentioned in connection with PMS symptoms. The results of a major new study provide a new perspective. According to this exciting research, a simple and inexpensive calcium supplement can dramatically reduce all the major symptoms of PMS. This discovery will undoubtedly lead to a reevaluation of our understanding of the causes of PMS, and spark a tremendous wave of interest in new research.

What Is Calcium?

Calcium is the most abundant mineral in your body. In fact, about 2½ pounds (or 1 kilogram) of calcium make up your bones and teeth. Calcium also plays an essential role in the transmission of nerve impulses, blood clotting, muscle contraction, and general cell activity.

What Is the Scientific Evidence for Calcium?

According to a large and well-designed study published in a 1998 issue of the *American Journal of Obstetrics and Gynecology*, calcium supplements are a simple and effective treatment for a wide variety of PMS symptoms. Dr. Susan Thys-Jacobs and colleagues of St. Luke's-Roosevelt Hospital Center in New York City authored this important study, the objective of which was to evaluate how well calcium supplements relieved the symptoms of PMS.

According to exciting new research, a simple and inexpensive calcium supplement can dramatically reduce all the major symptoms of PMS.

Dr. Thys-Jacobs had laid the groundwork for this study in earlier research. Several years earlier, she had been intrigued by the similarity between symptoms of PMS and the symptoms experienced by people with very low levels of calcium. If your calcium levels fall too low, you may feel agitated, irritable, and depressed, very much like how you feel during the time you experience PMS.[1] Furthermore, in 1995, Dr. Thys-Jacobs discovered that women with PMS have abnormally low levels of calcium at the time of ovulation, compared to the women without PMS.[2]

By itself, simply finding that women with PMS have low levels of calcium in the blood doesn't prove that calcium supplements will make PMS symptoms go away. Maybe PMS causes low calcium levels, rather than the reverse. However, back in 1989, Dr. Thys-Jacobs had already

PMS: Nature's Reminder to Get More Calcium?

Dr. Susan Thys-Jacobs, an endocrinologist and author of a major new study on calcium and PMS, recounts an experience from her practice. "One of my patients was on two kinds of antidepressants, and she was so miserable that GnRH inhibitors seemed to be her only choice." As you may recall from chapter 4, GnRH inhibitors are a last-resort treatment that essentially throw a woman into early menopause. But Thys-Jacobs found another option for her patient, and was able to report: "Calcium relieved her symptoms after only 2 months!"

According to Thys-Jacobs, the symptoms of PMS are nature's way of telling us to get more calcium. Whether her theory proves true or not, calcium is definitely a treatment with no downside. Calcium supplements are inexpensive and virtually harmless. They help prevent osteoporosis and, in general, are healthful for women anyway. Seldom do we find so simple a decision: Take calcium.

published the results of a small study that found calcium supplements effective in the treatment of PMS symptoms.[3] Other small studies had also reported similar results, although Dr. Thys-Jacobs's 1989 study involved too few participants to prove much.[4] Further evidence suggested that women with PMS are also at increased risk of later developing osteoporosis, for reasons that were not at all clear at the time.[5,6] Could it be that some problem with handling calcium is the cause of both PMS and osteoporosis?

Intrigued, Dr. Thys-Jacobs obtained funding for a large and definitive double-blind study to evaluate the use of calcium in PMS. The results, published in the *American Journal of Obstetrics and Gynecology* in 1998, provide unmistakable evidence that calcium is an effective treatment for PMS.

The 1998 Thys-Jacobs Study

This double-blind placebo-controlled trial followed 497 women for a period of three menstrual cycles.[7] Women taking part in the study were premenopausal and from 18 to 45 years of age. All were in generally good health and had regular menstrual cycles. Each woman was carefully screened prior to the study, to determine that she was regularly experiencing at least one of the following symptoms of premenstrual syndrome: mood swings, depression/sadness, tension/irritability, anxiety/nervousness, anger/aggression/ short temper, or crying spells. The women participating were selected from a variety of outpatient medical centers throughout the United States.

In order to ensure valid results, the researchers made sure that the placebo and the treatment groups were essentially identical on average with regard to ethnic background, age, weight, height, use of oral contraceptive, and length of menstrual cycle.

Women with PMS have abnormally low levels of calcium at the time of ovulation, compared to the women without PMS.

Approximately half the women were given a dose of calcium carbonate that provided 1,200 mg of calcium daily. (Calcium carbonate is one of the cheapest and most common types of calcium supplement.) The rest of the women were given a placebo. Both groups were treated for three menstrual cycles.

How Severe Is Your PMS?

Would you like to know how your PMS measures up? Here are the criteria Dr. Thys-Jacobs used in her calcium supplement study to measure the severity of the PMS of her study participants. Rate each symptom using the following scale: 0 for no symptoms; 1 for mild symptoms; 2 for moderate symptoms; and 3 for severe symptoms.

Emotional Symptoms

- Mood swings _____
- Depression/sadness _____
- Tension/irritability _____
- Anxiety/nervousness _____
- Anger/aggression/short temper _____
- Crying spells _____

Water Retention

- Swelling of extremities _____
- Tenderness, fullness of breasts _____
- Abdominal bloating _____

All participants were instructed to keep a diary, recording symptoms, side effects, other medications taken, and how well they followed the regime for taking their calcium (or placebo) treatments. During the study, participants were monitored every other week with telephone interviews, and monthly by follow-up visits.

In order to assess the extent of PMS symptoms, Thys-Jacobs and her fellow researchers used a numerical rating scale that evaluated 17 different symptoms, dividing them

Food Cravings

- Increased or decreased appetite _____
- Cravings for sweets or salts _____

Pain

- Abdominal cramping _____
- Generalized aches and pains _____
- Low back pain _____
- Headaches _____
- Fatigue _____
- Insomnia _____

If your total score is 0–17, you have no more than mild PMS; 18–34 indicates moderate PMS; and 35–51 indicates severe PMS.

into four categories: emotional symptoms, water retention, food cravings, and pain.

The results of this trial showed that calcium supplements were able to provide relief for a wide variety of PMS symptoms. The strongest results appeared during the third and final cycle of the study, suggesting that the effects of calcium supplements increase with continued use. By this time, women taking the calcium supplements showed a significant improvement of symptoms in all four

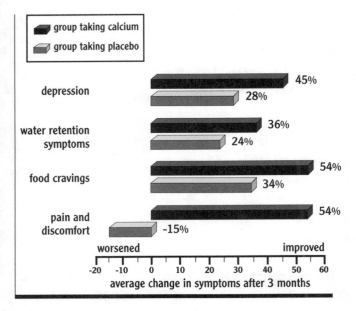

Figure 4. *Calcium supplements significantly reduced PMS symptoms.* (Thys-Jacobs S, et al., 1998.)

categories (see figure 4). The majority of women given calcium showed a significant improvement in PMS symptoms as defined by a 50% reduction in overall PMS symptom scores. As always happens in medical research, placebo treatment also reduced symptoms, but only in 36% of participants. From a mathematical point of view, there is no question that calcium was more effective than the placebo in this study.

A close look at the results tells us a great deal about how calcium supplements affect PMS. No improvement was seen in the first menstrual cycle, when women had been taking calcium for only a short time. This suggests that calcium levels in the body have to build up to reduce

PMS symptoms. During the second menstrual cycle, calcium produced benefits in all but one category (food cravings). By the end of the trial, calcium supplements had produced marked benefits in all but 2 of the 17 symptoms of PMS (insomnia and fatigue).

Of all the participants, only 8% of the women receiving calcium had no improvement or a worsening of symptoms, compared to 24% of the women taking the placebo. This means that three times as many women experienced no improvement or a worsening of symptoms with the placebo than with the calcium treatment. Again, this difference was mathematically significant.

This study provides concrete evidence that calcium is an effective treatment for PMS symptoms. It was large enough to provide mathematically meaningful results, and conducted and reported in a way that meets the highest scientific standards. The only element that's needed for calcium to be considered a proven treatment for PMS is confirmation by a different researcher.

How Do Calcium Supplements Help PMS?

The real answer to this question is: We really don't know. As described in chapter 3, this study has provoked a re-analysis of the causes of PMS. New theories are coming out in response to the Thys-Jacob study, and, by the time you read this, much more may be known than was available at press time. Anything stated at this time is very much still speculation.

How Calcium Compares with Conventional Treatments

Since there have been no studies that directly compare the effects of calcium to standard treatments for PMS, it is

What Makes a Good Scientific Study?

The 1998 Thys-Jacobs calcium study, designed to test the effectiveness of calcium as a treatment for PMS, is a good example of what it takes to design a meaningful study. In any research, the more people studied, the more likely the research is to yield accurate results. With nearly 500 participants, the Thys-Jacobs study was adequately large. It represented a good cross-section of the general population in ethnicity, average age, height and weight, as well as other factors related to the study, such as average length of menstrual cycle.

This important study was also double-blind: Neither the subjects nor the doctors knew who was getting the real treatment or who was receiving the fake treatment, or placebo. The placebo group is important to any study because people are

not possible to make any reliable statement about its relative effectiveness. However, we can say that, compared to standard treatments for PMS, calcium is both side-effect free and very inexpensive.

In the Thys-Jacobs study, calcium did not seem to produce any side effects. Or, to be more precise, it didn't produce significantly more side effects than the placebo. Participants in both the placebo and calcium groups reported a variety of minor problems—primarily headache, nasal stuffiness, and overall pain. Because they occurred in both groups, they were almost certainly not due to the treatment, but merely happened on their own or were caused by the power of suggestion.

In contrast, standard treatments for PMS can cause many side effects. Prozac can cause an inability to achieve known to feel better simply because they take something they *believe* is a medicine. The placebo group helps determine how much of the benefits might be the result of believing you are getting better and how much is due to the treatment itself. Also, the placebo group provides a way to compare the results from those who were given the treatment to a "control" group who are left untreated (or given a placebo).

Because the 1998 Thys-Jacobs study met these important criteria, we can say that its results provided strong evidence that calcium supplements can effectively treat a wide variety of PMS symptoms. In view of its safety, cost, and general helpfulness, calcium will very likely become the predominant treatment for PMS.

orgasm, along with nausea and insomnia; birth control pills can cause blood clots, weight gain, headaches, cramps; antianxiety medications such as Valium can cause drowsiness, confusion, and fatigue; and GnRH-blocking drugs (and to a lesser extent Danocrine) essentially cause menopause to begin. Compared to these treatments, calcium stands alone.

Calcium is also far cheaper than conventional treatment. If you shop around and don't insist on getting a chewable product, you can obtain a month's supply of calcium carbonate for under $10. This isn't surprising, since calcium carbonate is simply limestone. In comparison, conventional treatments can easily cost more than a $100 per month.

Finally, calcium is just plain good for you. It is very likely that all women should take calcium supplements simply on general principle. In fact, calcium sounds so good that it is amazing its value for PMS wasn't discovered long ago.

Dosage

The optimum dose of calcium for reducing PMS symptoms is not completely clear, but the Thys-Jacobs study suggests that 1,200 mg daily is appropriate.

Calcium comes in many forms, each with its own pros and cons. Calcium carbonate, as used in the Thys-Jacobs study, is one of the most inexpensive and convenient forms of calcium. However, some women have trouble absorbing it. Taking it with meals should help, because the stomach acid released during a meal helps to dissolve it.

Calcium supplements from bone meal and oyster shell are also inexpensive, but may contain lead.

Calcium citrate is generally better absorbed than other forms of calcium. However, it is more expensive and you have to take quite a few (and usually quite large) pills to get enough calcium.

Orange juice, soy milk, and rice milk are often forti-

It is fair to say that, compared to standard treatments for PMS, calcium is both side-effect free and inexpensive.

fied with calcium citrate malate, a special form of calcium that is highly absorbable, and has been proven to help osteoporosis. (For more information on osteoporosis, see *The Natural Pharmacist Guide to Menopause*.)

In order to absorb calcium, you need to have enough vitamin D in your body (which is why vitamin D is added to milk). Your body can synthesize vitamin D when the skin is exposed to the sun, but if you stay indoors much of the time or wear sunblock when you go out, taking 400 IU of vitamin D daily along with your calcium may be a good idea. (For more information on vitamin D, see *The Natural Pharmacist: Your Complete Guide to Vitamins and Supplements.*)

Safety Issues

Although there is no reason to take more than 1,200 mg a day, in general, an intake of 2,000 mg of calcium or less daily is considered safe.[8] However, if you have cancer, hyperparathyroidism, or sarcoidosis, you should only take calcium under the supervision of a physician.

People with kidney stones or a history of kidney stones are often cautioned not to take supplemental calcium. The reason for this warning is that kidney stones are commonly made of calcium oxalate crystals. Recent studies, however, failed to find a relationship between increased calcium intake and the occurrence of kidney stones.[9] In fact, some studies show that the risk for kidney stones actually goes down with the use of calcium.[10] Whether or not calcium plays a preventive role in kidney stones, these studies certainly cast doubt on the long-held belief that people who form kidney stones shouldn't take calcium. Check with your physician for the latest information.

Vitamin D is safe when taken at 400 IU daily, but can be toxic when taken at dosages higher than 1,000 IU daily. Individuals with sarcoidosis or hyperparathyroidism should not take vitamin D except on medical advice.

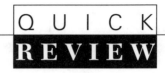

QUICK
REVIEW

- Important new research provides strong evidence that calcium supplements dramatically reduce a wide variety of PMS symptoms, including depression, anxiety, crying spells, breast pain and other water retention symptoms, food cravings, headaches, and general aches and pains.

- Evidence suggests that the effects of calcium supplements increase with continued use.

- Compared to many conventional medications, calcium supplements are inexpensive, safe, effective, and free of side effects. They are also good for you!

- Although the optimum dose of calcium is not clear, 1,200 mg daily is suggested as appropriate.

- Many forms of calcium are available. Calcium carbonate (taken with meals for best results) may be the most practical. Orange juice and other beverages are now commonly fortified with a highly absorbable form of calcium called calcium citrate malate.

- Taking vitamin D supplements at 400 IU daily will ensure that you can absorb the calcium you take.

- Although calcium and vitamin D are considered safe, if you have cancer, hyperparathyroidism, or sarcoidosis, you should only take calcium and/or vitamin D under the supervision of a physician. Vitamin D should not be taken in dosages higher than 1,000 IU daily.

Chasteberry

A Popular European Treatment for PMS

T he herb chasteberry, often referred to by its Latin name *Vitex agnus-castus* or simply vitex, is widely used in Germany as a treatment for PMS symptoms. Although the scientific evidence for chasteberry is not yet strong, so many German physicians regard it as the primary treatment for PMS that here it will have a chapter of its own.

What Is Chasteberry?

The chasteberry plant is a member of the verbena family. It is sometimes known as the "chaste tree," even though it is more a shrub than a tree. Chasteberry is commonly found on riverbanks and nearby foothills in central Asia and around the Mediterranean. It was carried across the Atlantic, and has "gone native" throughout much of the southeastern United States.

Perhaps the most noticeable feature of this plant is its purple flowers (see figure 5). After the bloom fades, a dark

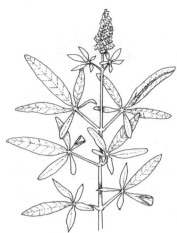

Figure 5. *Chasteberry*

brown, peppercorn-size fruit develops, with a pleasant odor that might remind you of peppermint. When dried, this fruit becomes medicinal chasteberry, which is used to treat PMS.

The fruit of the chasteberry has a pleasant odor reminiscent of peppermint. When dried, this fruit becomes medicinal chasteberry, used to treat PMS.

The Roman historian Pliny (A.D. 23–79) reported that chasteberry was used for a variety of menstrual ailments.[1] However, the modern medicinal use of chasteberry for PMS dates back only to the 1950s, when a German pharmaceutical firm first produced a standardized extract of chasteberry. Since then, this herb has become a standard European treatment for PMS, as well as for menstrual irregularities and infertility.

What Is Chasteberry Used for Today?

For many German physicians, chasteberry is the first treatment to try when a woman complains of PMS symptoms, and Germany's official herb regulatory agency, the Commission E, has approved the use of chasteberry to treat premenstrual complaints.[2,3]

What Is the Scientific Evidence for Chasteberry?

In a rather informal study enrolling a total of more than 1,500 women with PMS, doctors rated chasteberry as effective about 90% of the time.[4,5] Women reported significant or complete improvement in such symptoms as breast pain, fluid retention, headache, and fatigue. However, this study did not involve a placebo control group, and all participants knew they were being treated. Therefore, the results are more a survey of physician experiences with chasteberry than actual scientific evidence.

Although the opinion of physicians is meaningful, it is definitely not proof. Decades of experience have shown us how easily even seasoned professionals can overestimate or underestimate the effectiveness of a treatment, based on their preconceptions and the power of suggestion. When it comes to medical treatments, well-designed scientific studies are required to produce dependable evidence.

Unfortunately, the research record for chasteberry is still weak. A search of the medical

The Roman historian Pliny (A.D. 23–79) reported that chasteberry was used for a variety of menstrual ailments.

Jill's Story

Jill's chief PMS complaints centered on fluid retention and tiredness. Jill, who is 5 feet, 5 inches tall and 121 pounds, says, "When it's bad, I feel like I weigh a ton. All of my body aches, and I just feel exhausted. Not depressed really, just dragged down. It's hard to describe."

Under the advice of a naturopathic physician, she started taking an alcohol extract of chasteberry. The schedule called for 200 mg daily, starting with day 14 of her cycle and ending when the period stopped.

After a couple of months, Jill noticed significant improvement in all her symptoms. "It's not exactly like my body is jumping for joy," she says, "but instead of overwhelming me, my fatigue is just annoying. I'd say there's a 75% improvement."

literature conducted during the writing of this book failed to find any double-blind placebo-controlled studies that directly evaluated the benefits of chasteberry for PMS symptoms.

One double-blind study has been performed; unfortunately, it compared chasteberry against vitamin B_6 (pyridoxine) instead of placebo.[6] Published in 1997, this study followed 175 women given either a standardized chasteberry extract or 200 mg of vitamin B_6 daily.

Chasteberry proved at least as effective as vitamin B_6. Both treatments produced significant improvements in all major symptoms of PMS, including breast tenderness, edema, tension, headache, and depression.

Although this study has been widely described as proof that chasteberry is effective for PMS, it doesn't ac-

Unfortunately, from the point of view of evaluating the evidence, Jill was not taking just chasteberry. She was also taking "a big spoonful, give or take" of flaxseed oil every day (not just during the second half of her cycle) and a vitamin supplement containing B vitamin complex, magnesium, zinc, and vitamins C, E, and A. Keeping these additional factors in mind (not to mention the power of suggestion), it's difficult to say how much of the improvement she felt stemmed from using this particular herb. We need properly designed studies to know for sure. In chapter 9, we'll see how another herb, ginkgo, might also help fluid retention related to PMS.

tually prove anything at all. As we'll see in chapter 8, vitamin B_6 itself has not been proven effective for PMS. Therefore, the fact that chasteberry works just as well as vitamin B_6 establishes little.

Patients given chasteberry in this study did report improvement in PMS symptoms, However, without a control group it's impossible to determine how much of the improvement was due to the placebo effect alone. It is a known fact that placebo treatment is highly effective for PMS. For example, in one study, women with PMS who were given placebo showed a 70% improvement in symptoms.[7] Therefore, we really need a good, large-scale, double-blind placebo-controlled study to discover just how effective chasteberry really is—beyond the inevitable effects of suggestion.

How Does Chasteberry Work?

Research has shown that, unlike some other herbs used for women's health problems, chasteberry does not contain any plant equivalent of estrogen or progesterone. Rather, it acts on the pituitary gland to suppress the release of a hormone called prolactin.[8–12]

> **By diminishing prolactin levels, chasteberry may reduce breast tenderness.**

Prolactin is a hormone that naturally rises during pregnancy to stimulate milk production. As mentioned in chapter 3, prolactin levels may also rise in PMS, causing breast tenderness and perhaps other symptoms as well. By diminishing prolactin levels, chasteberry may reduce these symptoms.

Interestingly, because elevated prolactin levels can also cause infertility, chasteberry is sometimes tried as a fertility drug.[13] If you don't want to get pregnant, keep this in mind!

Chasteberry also appears to increase progesterone levels, either directly or indirectly, through the influence of reduced prolactin. By affecting progesterone and prolactin, chasteberry can normalize the second half of the menstrual cycle (the luteal phase).[14] As described in chapter 2, this is the interval during which PMS symptoms occur.

What Is in Chasteberry?

Although we can identify a number of compounds present in the fruit of the chasteberry, we don't know which one (or ones) helps relieve premenstrual symptoms. Two of the most studied constituents, agnoside and aucubin, belong to a family of substances known as iridoid glycosides. However, chasteberry contains many other unique substances as well, such as viticin, casticin and castine.[15–18] Thus far, no individual ingredient in chasteberry has been found to produce the same effects as does the whole.

Dosage

Because we can choose from so many different chasteberry products on the market, giving general dosage guidelines is difficult. I recommend following the specific directions on the label. Unlike most herbs, chasteberry is usually taken only once daily.

Physicians report that chasteberry usually begins to work within about 3 to 4 weeks, but full effects may not develop for months.[19,20]

Safety Issues

Comprehensive toxicity studies of chasteberry have not been performed. However, in studies involving thousands of women, the use of chasteberry has not been associated with any serious adverse effects.[21,22] Mild side effects occasionally reported by those using chasteberry include nausea, headache, and allergic skin reactions. One case reported a woman whose ovary produced multiple eggs at one time, apparently due to chasteberry.[23] The same effect is sometimes seen with fertility drugs, but whether chasteberry really caused it in this case is not clear.

Because chasteberry lowers the milk-producing hormone prolactin, this herb is definitely not an appropriate treatment

Interestingly, because elevated prolactin levels can also cause infertility, chasteberry is sometimes tried as a fertility drug.

for pregnant or nursing women. Furthermore, the herb's safety in adolescents and in those with severe liver or kidney disorders has not been established. Although no known drug interactions have been reported with chasteberry, it is possible that this herb could interfere with hormonal medications such as estrogen, progesterone, or the drug bromocriptine (a pharmaceutical that reduces prolactin levels).

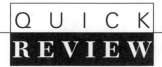

QUICK REVIEW

- The herb chasteberry, also known as vitex or *Vitex agnus-castus,* is widely used in Germany to treat the symptoms of PMS.

- Open studies suggest that chasteberry is effective for about 90% of women. It seems to start working within about 3 to 4 weeks, but may take much longer to reach its full effect. However, good double-blind studies have not yet been conducted.

- Chasteberry appears to work by inhibiting the secretion of the hormone prolactin.

- The proper dose of chasteberry, which is usually taken only once a day, varies with specific products.

- Chasteberry seldom causes any side effects, but researchers have not yet performed full formal safety studies. Chasteberry should not be used by pregnant or nursing women.

Evening Primrose Oil and Essential Fatty Acids

Many women experience breast tenderness and pain as part of PMS. These episodes are known officially as *cyclic mastalgia* (mastalgia means "painful breast"), *cyclic mastitis* (mastitis means "inflamed breast"), or sometimes *fibrocystic breast disease.* Your symptoms may range from an uncomfortable feeling of fullness in your breasts to a pain that is severe enough to disrupt your life. At its worst, cyclic mastalgia can interfere with your sleep, your sexual relationships, and your ability to carry out your daily activities.

Julia's story illustrates just how disturbing cyclic mastalgia can be.

When the tenderness in her breast increased to the point of actual pain, Julia turned to her doctor. She had dreaded this appointment. Even though she knew that breast cancer was usually painless, her imagination ran wild, and she was close to tears. After a careful exam, the doctor asked her to sit down. "This is it," she thought.

"Does this pain come and go?" her doctor asked. The question took her by surprise. "Is it worse at one particular time of the month?" he repeated.

Although Julia had never thought about it, she suddenly realized that the pain *did* seem to be worse at certain times of the month. In fact, she might even go a few weeks without any discomfort at all. Her doctor listened patiently as she explained.

Evening primrose oil is an accepted treatment in Europe and North America for PMS breast pain.

"I'm thinking that this tenderness has something to do with premenstrual syndrome," he said with a gentle smile. "I don't feel anything that would make me think breast cancer, but we'll schedule you for a mammogram just in case. Once it comes back negative, as I'm sure it will, we'll work on finding something to help you with your discomfort."

As predicted, the mammogram came back without a hint of breast cancer. Her physician suggested she try evening primrose oil. "It may take a month or two before you feel the effects, but it seems to work. There are several drugs that can do the same thing, but evening primrose is safer than any of them, and I'd like you to try it first."

Evening primrose oil (EPO) is a safe natural product and is now an accepted treatment in Europe and North America for the cyclic breast pain of PMS. Doctors sometimes recommend it for other PMS symptoms, too, but evening primrose oil is probably most useful for relieving breast discomfort.

What Is Evening Primrose Oil?

Evening primrose, a native American wildflower, was named because its brilliant yellow flowers open only in the

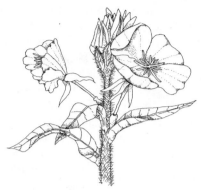

Figure 6. *Evening primrose*

late afternoon or early evening hours (see figure 6). Once it was found exclusively in eastern North America, but now evening primrose grows throughout Europe, North America, and even in parts of Asia.

Botanists know the evening primrose as *Oenothera biennis.* Its other, less commonly used, names include Night Willow Herb, King's Cure-All, and Fever Plant. The fatty seeds of the evening primrose yield an oil that is a rich natural source of *gamma-linolenic acid* (GLA). GLA is an *essential fatty acid.* Scientists think that GLA is the key ingredient in evening primrose oil that relieves PMS breast discomfort. Other natural sources of GLA include borage oil and black currant oil. Though borage and black currant oils may also be effective, fewer scientific studies have focused on them than on evening primrose oil.

The Importance of Essential Fatty Acids

You may think that all fats are bad for you, but this is not the case with essential fatty acids (EFAs). Unlike the many fats we try to avoid, essential fatty acids are as important to our good health as vitamins. Since our bodies can't manufacture them, we need to get these fatty acids from our diet.

There are two major families of essential fatty acids: the omega-6 and the omega-3 fatty acids. Both types are

Essential fatty acids are as important to our good health as vitamins.

found in food, but some foods contain higher levels than others. Foods that are rich in omega-6 fatty acids include mother's milk, seed and vegetable oils, organ meats, and most kinds of nuts. Good sources of omega-3 fatty acids are green leafy vegetables and coldwater fish, such as salmon and mackerel. Omega-3 fatty acids are the more famous of the two types, due to evidence that they can help prevent heart disease. Yet omega-6 fatty acids also seem to offer health benefits.

Normally, we don't eat foods that contain much GLA. Yet there is a way that we can get enough GLA in our diet: by eating foods that contain another EFA, called linoleic acid. Our bodies can then convert the linoleic acid to GLA. However, as I will soon explain, women with PMS-related breast pain may have trouble carrying out this conversion.

What Are the Benefits of Evening Primrose Oil in PMS?

Evidence suggests that evening primrose oil (EPO) can relieve the symptoms of breast discomfort that often accompany PMS. Over several months, it appears to significantly reduce symptoms in almost half of the women who use it. Not only that, it is practically free of side effects.

EPO is also used to treat other conditions, such as eczema and diabetic neuropathy. (See *The Natural Phar-*

macist: Your Complete Guide to Herbs for more information on this useful natural treatment.)

What Is the Scientific Evidence for EPO?

The Cardiff Mastalgia Clinic at the University of Wales (Great Britain) has provided much of what we know about evening primrose oil. This clinic began its work in 1973 and continues to pioneer both the research and the treatment of mastalgia. Doctors at this center have refined our understanding of cyclic mastalgia and have provided long-term care for thousands of women with cyclic breast pain.

The Cardiff Clinic physicians regularly experiment with different treatments for cyclic breast pain and then record the outcome. While definitely less formal than a proper double-blind study (see Double-Blind Studies later in this chapter) this type of information can give us real insight into the effectiveness of a treatment.

One report published by a physician at the Cardiff Clinic in 1985 compares four different therapies for women with severe, painful mastalgia: EPO and the pharmaceuticals danazol (the generic form of Danocrine), bromocriptine, and progestins (often but not quite accurately

Evidence suggests that evening primrose oil can relieve breast discomfort that often accompanies PMS.

called progesterone).[1] All the women involved in the study had suffered from cyclic breast pain for at least 6 months and for at least 10 days of each menstrual cycle.

The treatment was given for 3 to 6 months and then either stopped or reduced. If the pain returned, each woman resumed the same treatment if her response had

Randi's Story

Randi never expected PMS to interfere with her new-found resolve to lose weight. After months of eating better and taking aerobics classes, Randi felt good about herself for the first time in years.

However, she encountered one obstacle. For nearly half of every month, she couldn't exercise. For years, she'd felt breast discomfort with her monthly cycle. It had never been more than an annoyance. But now all the painful bouncing and jumping of aerobics was unbearable. It seemed more like torture than exercise.

Randi was afraid her classmates thought she was flaky, coming for a few weeks and then disappearing for just as long. Finally even her instructor asked about it. Hesitantly, Randi explained her problem. To her surprise, the instructor knew immediately what she was talking about.

been good, or started on another treatment if her response had not been good.

According to clinic records, EPO was effective in 47% of participants. This was about the same rate of effectiveness as seen among women given the drug bromocriptine. Danazol was a bit more effective, producing significant benefits in 70% of participants. Progestins were not beneficial.

Regarding side effects, however, evening primrose oil was clearly superior. Bromocriptine produced significant side effects in 33% of the participants (primarily nausea, headaches, and dizziness) and danazol caused problems for 22% (disturbance of their menstrual cycles, headache,

"I have the same problem," the instructor said. "Or at least I used to." She then told Randi about evening primrose oil and how it helped her to continue teaching classes throughout the month. "I also wear a good support bra," she said. Just to be sure, Randi first checked with her doctor. He, too, confirmed that evening primrose oil might relieve her painful breasts. He cautioned her not to expect immediate results, as it usually took several months for evening primrose oil to even *begin* to help. "It might take as long as 6 to 8 months," he told her, "for you to feel the maximum benefits. But be patient. This is not folk medicine. It's even recommended in my official AMA Drug Evaluations manual.[2] It really works."

Nine months later, a happier and thinner Randi was pleased to recommend evening primrose to a new aerobics classmate who was having the same problem.

nausea, and weight gain). In comparison, the side effects from evening primrose oil were minimal. Only 2% of the women complained of any side effects, and it was just "a bloated feeling with vague nausea."

Despite the higher success rate of danazol, the Cardiff Clinic concluded that evening primrose oil provided the best first-line treatment for cyclic mastalgia.[3] Women accepted EPO more easily, the clinic said, because its side effects were so rare and because women preferred to avoid "hormonal" treatments.

The Longmore Breast Unit at the Royal Infirmary of Edinburgh also reported good results with EPO.[4]

Double-Blind Studies

Although these results are impressive, they are relatively informal. To really know whether a treatment is effective, you need double-blind placebo-controlled studies that completely eliminate the power of suggestion. (See the description of this type of study, and the reasons for them, in chapter 4.) One such study was reported in 1981. This double-blind placebo-controlled trial followed 73 women suffering from cyclic mastalgia.[5] The results were consistent with the Cardiff clinic report: EPO reduced pain in almost 50% of the women, compared to a reduction of pain in only 19% of the women taking a placebo.

However, this study was reported in only a very brief form, and many details are missing. We need better-designed and better-reported studies to know for sure how effective EPO actually is in relieving cyclic mastalgia.

What About PMS in General?

We find the same lack of good studies when we look for evidence of EPO's benefit for general PMS symptoms. A review of the literature, published in 1996, found only five placebo-controlled studies with enough published information to enable us to evaluate their meaningfulness.[6] Most of these had serious problems in their reporting or design, and the two best-designed studies found no difference between the effectiveness of evening primrose oil and placebo treatment.[7,8] One study that *did* find positive results failed to analyze them mathematically to see if they were significant.[9] Another study found that EPO helps PMS-related depression but provided no other benefits overall.[10]

The bottom line is that evening primrose oil is probably not terribly effective for treating PMS as a whole. It is best used to relieve cyclic mastalgia.

How Do EPO and EFAs Work in Cyclic Mastalgia?

Essential fatty acids play a major role in pain and inflammation. Studies show that abnormal levels of essential fatty acids are found in the bodies of women who suffer from premenstrual breast pain.[11] A close look at the data from these studies revealed that these women were getting enough essential fatty acids in their diet, but they were unable to convert them properly to GLA. This problem may cause inflammation in the breasts (as well as elsewhere). Essential fatty acids can also affect the action of various hormones that we believe play a role in breast tenderness, including prolactin, estrogen, progesterone, and angiotensin. I've already discussed the first three of these hormones in previous chapters. Chasteberry is known to reduce prolactin release; danazol, birth control pills, and GnRH inhibitors all affect estrogen and progesterone levels. Angiotensin is another important hormone in the body that can dramatically influence fluid retention, another classic PMS symptom.

However, much of this remains scientific speculation. More research is needed before we can come to any definite conclusion about how EPO affects cyclic mastalgia.

Dosage

To relieve the cyclic breast discomfort and pain of PMS, take 2 to 4 g of evening primrose oil daily, with food. Remember that it may be 1 to 2 months before you begin to feel the benefits and 6 to 8 months for EPO to reach its full effects. So be patient.

Borage oil and black currant oil also contain high levels of GLA and may help cyclic mastitis. However, they are not identical to evening primrose and may not work as well.

Safety Issues

Evening primrose oil is a very safe substance. Animal studies suggest that evening primrose oil is completely nontoxic and noncarcinogenic.[12,13,14] Over 4,000 people

Evening primrose oil is a very safe substance.

have participated in trials of GLA, primarily in the form of evening primrose oil, and they experienced no significant adverse effects.[15,16,17] While somewhat less than 2% of the people who take evening primrose oil complain of headaches, mild gastrointestinal distress, or both, in most double-blind studies of EPO there were no significant differences in the rate of side effects between the treated group and the placebo group. In addition, over 500,000 prescriptions of EPO had been issued by the U.K. National Health Service by 1992, with no definite reports of linked negative effects.

Early case reports suggested that the GLA present in evening primrose oil might worsen a special form of epilepsy known as temporal lobe epilepsy, and also bipolar disorder (manic depression), but later reports have not confirmed this.[18]

A maximum safe dose of EPO for children, pregnant or nursing mothers, or those with severe liver or kidney disease has not been established.

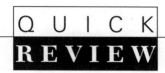

- Evening primrose oil is a safe natural product that has become an accepted treatment for the painful breasts of PMS, known as *cyclic mastalgia*.
- Evidence suggests that over a period of several months, evening primrose oil can significantly reduce breast pain in almost 50% of women who use it.
- Evening primrose oil is probably not very effective for PMS in general.
- The proper dosage is 2 to 4 g daily, with food.
- Evening primrose oil is safe and free of significant side effects.

Other Food Supplements for PMS

In addition to calcium, herbs, and evening primrose oil, other vitamins and minerals may also help your PMS symptoms. Double-blind studies suggest that a standard multivitamin and multimineral tablet can reduce your PMS discomfort, most likely by improving your overall nutrition. Vitamin E is best known as an antioxidant that can lessen your risk of heart disease, but when taken alone, it may relieve your PMS symptoms as well. Preliminary studies suggest that the mineral magnesium may improve PMS-related mood changes and fluid congestion, and it may offer the additional benefit of preventing migraine headaches.

Ironically, although vitamin B_6 is widely accepted by conventional physicians in both Europe and North America, it doesn't seem to work on PMS. Nonetheless, taking any of these treatments, you are in a "win–win" situation. Regardless of whether or not they improve PMS symptoms, they are good for your overall health.

Multivitamin/Mineral Supplements: Can Reduce Many PMS Symptoms

Instead of purchasing a lot of individual supplements, it's cheaper for you to buy one capsule or tablet that contains a bit of everything. According to double-blind studies enrolling about 350 women, not only is this good insurance against deficiencies in your diet, but it may reduce your PMS symptoms.[1–4]

In one of the largest of these studies, 223 women randomly received either full doses of a multivitamin and mineral supplement, low doses of the same supplement, or placebo for three menstrual cycles.[5] The results showed significant improvement in PMS symptoms among the women in the full-dose group as compared to the low-dose or placebo groups.

None of these studies tell us which vitamins and minerals are most helpful in relieving PMS symptoms. Still, how can you go wrong taking a multivitamin? Most of us don't eat all the types of food that we should. If we improve our general nutrition, this will undoubtedly help all of our health problems.

In the remainder of this chapter, I will discuss specific nutrients that may help PMS symptoms.

Vitamin E: May Reduce PMS Symptoms and Protect Against Heart Disease and Cancer

Vitamin E is most famous as an *antioxidant,* a substance that can neutralize the dangerous chemicals in our bodies known as *free radicals.* Free radicals damage cells throughout our bodies and play a role in the development of many illnesses, including cancer, heart disease, cataracts, and arthritis. Good evidence tells us that regular

Nancy's Story

Nancy cured her PMS symptoms accidentally. At her regular visit to the gynecologist, the physician asked Nancy questions about her diet. When she heard Nancy's answers, she shook her head. "You seem to live mostly on pasta and chocolate," she said. "That's not really good enough."

Nancy explained calmly that she couldn't stand fruits and vegetables and simply wasn't going to eat them. "At 38 years old I know myself well enough, and I know that I'm not going to change."

"What about vitamins?" the doctor asked. It turned out that Nancy had no objection to these. "But I'm not taking 20 pills a day. About 3 pills is probably all I can handle." The physician recommended a multivitamin and mineral supplement that contained extra high doses of vitamin E. She also suggested a

use of vitamin E can reduce the risk of heart disease and certain forms of cancer (for more information on heart disease, see *The Natural Pharmacist Guide to Heart Disease Prevention*).

What Is the Scientific Evidence for Vitamin E?

Three double-blind studies performed by the same researcher suggest that vitamin E can also improve many symptoms of PMS.[6,7,8] The largest of these studies was a double-blind trial that followed 75 women between 18 and 45 years of age.[9] Participants were randomly assigned either placebo or doses of vitamin E at 150, 300, or 600 IU (international units) per day. The study found that vitamin E (at all doses) was more effective than placebo in re-separate extra calcium supplement, since, as she explained, "you can't fit enough calcium into a multivitamin."

Nancy was quite religious about taking her supplements. "Considering how I eat," she said, "it's the least I can do for myself." Her doctor had told her not to expect any obvious benefit. "These supplements are for the long term," she said.

But in that, the doctor was wrong. Within two menstrual cycles, Nancy noticed that something was missing. It was her PMS; the symptoms she'd lived with for decades were gone.

Was it the calcium? The vitamin E? Or some combination of nutrients? We don't know; better scientific studies are necessary before we can make any ultimate recommendations. But Nancy is the beneficiary of better nutrition in any case.

lieving mood swings, irritability, nervous tension, anxiety, headaches, fatigue, appetite disturbances, dizziness, depression, crying, and insomnia.

Dosage
The typical recommended dosage of vitamin E is 400 IU daily. This dosage should be sufficient to provide the heart protective effects of vitamin E as well.

Safety Issues
Vitamin E at a dosage of 400 IU daily is believed to be safe. However, because vitamin E "thins" the blood slightly, it should not be combined with strong blood-thinning medications such as Coumadin (warfarin), heparin,

or even possibly aspirin except on medical advice. It is also conceivable that vitamin E might interact with natural substances that mildly thin the blood, such as the herbs garlic and ginkgo.

Magnesium: May Be Helpful for PMS Depression

According to some writers on natural medicine, the mineral magnesium is one of the most important supplements to consider when treating PMS.[10] Magnesium plays an essential role in hundreds of enzyme reactions throughout our bodies, including those that produce energy.[11] Magnesium also helps control the passage of minerals such as sodium, potassium, and calcium in and out of cells.

According to some writers on natural medicine, magnesium is one of the most important supplements to consider when treating PMS.

Most of us could benefit nutritionally by taking a little extra magnesium. In one survey of 27,000 Americans, only 25% had enough magnesium in their diet.[12] Whether or not magnesium supplements help your PMS, they will improve your health in other ways.

What Is the Scientific Evidence for Magnesium?

One small double-blind trial suggests that magnesium can lessen PMS depression.[13]

Another small double-blind preliminary study found that regular use of magnesium could reduce symptoms of PMS-related fluid retention.[14]

Finally, a double-blind study of 81 people found that magnesium (at a dosage of 600 mg daily) can significantly reduce the chances of developing a migraine headache.[15] While this study did not specifically examine women with PMS-related migraines, it certainly suggests that the mineral might help.

Dosage

A good dosage of magnesium for maintaining your general health is 250 to 350 mg daily. If you are using it for PMS symptoms, though, you could try a much larger dosage of 1,000 mg daily, beginning on the 15th day of your menstrual cycle and continuing until the onset of your period.

Some nutritionally oriented physicians believe that magnesium works best when combined with vitamin B_6.[16] Out of the many available forms of magnesium, the best may be magnesium citrate, aspartate, succinate, or fumarate.

Magnesium may be able to improve many symptoms of PMS, including mood changes, fluid retention, and possibly even migraine headaches.

Safety Issues

The dosage of magnesium supplementation I recommend for PMS symptoms is higher than that needed for good nutrition, but it should be safe for healthy women. However, if you have any chronic medical problems (particularly heart or kidney disease) or take any medications regularly, you should definitely check with your physician first. Some forms of magnesium, especially magnesium sulfate, chloride, or hydroxide, may cause diarrhea. Magnesium supplements may also reduce the absorption of calcium.

The maximum safe doses for children and pregnant or nursing women have not been established.

Vitamin B$_6$: Widely Recommended, but May Not Be Effective

Vitamin B$_6$ is also known as pyridoxine. This water-soluble vitamin is required for more than 60 enzymes to function properly in your body. (Enzymes are chemicals that speed up the rate of reaction in our cells.) Vitamin B$_6$ also helps reduce levels of homocysteine, a substance found in the blood that is believed to accelerate heart disease.

> **It is definitely beneficial to your health to get enough vitamin B$_6$ in your diet. However, it may not help PMS symptoms.**

Vitamin B$_6$ is essential to human nutrition, but many Americans are not getting enough of it in their diets. A survey of 11,658 adults found that 71% of men and 90% of women were deficient in vitamin B$_6$.[17] In elderly people, vitamin B$_6$ is the most commonly deficient water-soluble vitamin, and children don't get enough of it, either.[18,19]

It is definitely beneficial to your health to get enough vitamin B$_6$ in your diet. However, despite many claims to the contrary, vitamin B$_6$ does not appear to help PMS symptoms.

What Is the Scientific Evidence for Vitamin B$_6$?

A recent properly designed double-blind trial of 120 women who had PMS found that vitamin B$_6$ was ineffective.[20] In this study, three prescription antidepressants were compared against vitamin B$_6$ (300 mg daily) and placebo. All the participants received 3 months of real treatment and 3 months of placebo. While the antidepressants worked well, vitamin B_6 proved to be no better than placebo.

Before this study, there had been about 12 scientific trials investigating the effects of vitamin B_6 on PMS. Though all were double-blind and placebo-controlled, only one involved enough women to be meaningful, and all of the studies suffered from significant design flaws.[21] Furthermore, only three studies even suggested that vitamin B_6 can improve PMS symptoms; the others had either inconclusive results or they found no benefit at all.

While some books on natural medicine try to explain away the negative results by claiming that too little vitamin B_6 was used in the studies, there was actually no correlation between dosage and effectiveness. The bottom line is that vitamin B_6, though it contributes to your general good health, will apparently not help your PMS symptoms.

Dosage

Many nutritionally oriented physicians recommend taking 25 to 50 mg of vitamin B_6 daily.

Safety Issues

Vitamin B_6 appears to be completely safe for adults when taken in doses up to 50 mg a day. However, if you take more than 2,000 mg (2 g) daily, you will run a severe risk of developing nerve damage. Nerve-related symptoms have even been reported at doses as low as 200 mg when taken for a long period of time.[22,23] There have also been a few reports of liver inflammation when vitamin B_6 was taken in quantities of more than 50 mg in one dose.[24]

Maximum safe doses of vitamin B_6 for children, pregnant or nursing women, or those with Parkinson's disease or severe liver or kidney disease have not been established.

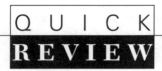

- Double-blind studies involving over 350 people suggest that multivitamin/mineral tablets can improve your PMS symptoms as well as your overall nutrition.

- Vitamin E is an antioxidant best known for its ability to reduce the risk of heart disease and some forms of cancer, but a few double-blind studies suggest that it can reduce PMS symptoms as well. The typical recommended dosage is 400 IU daily.

- Magnesium is an essential dietary mineral, but most Americans do not consume enough of it. Preliminary evidence suggests that it can improve PMS-related mood changes, symptoms of fluid retention, and perhaps PMS migraines. For general health, a good daily dosage is 250 to 350 mg; for PMS symptoms you can take 1,000 mg daily beginning on the 15th day of your menstrual cycle and continuing until the onset of your period. Please consult your doctor before taking magnesium if you have any chronic medical problems.

- Although high doses of vitamin B_6 are widely used to treat the symptoms of PMS, they are probably not effective. However, since most Americans don't get enough vitamin B_6 in their diets, taking nutritional (low-dose) supplements is probably a good idea.

Other Herbs
Used for PMS

We've already discussed the use of chasteberry and evening primrose oil for PMS. This chapter discusses other options that might be helpful. These include *Ginkgo biloba* (never traditionally used to treat PMS symptoms, but found to be surprisingly effective in a double-blind study) and black cohosh and dong quai, both of which have a long history of use for PMS symptoms, but no scientific evidence to back them.

Ginkgo biloba: Seems to Relieve PMS Fluid Retention

Traceable back 300 million years, the ginkgo (*Ginkgo biloba* L.) is the oldest surviving species of tree. Although it died out in Europe during the Ice Ages, ginkgo survived in China, Japan, and other parts of East Asia. It has been cultivated extensively for both ceremonial and medical purposes, and some particularly revered trees have been lovingly tended for over 1,000 years. Presently, a special

extract of ginkgo leaf (see figure 7) is the most widely prescribed herb product in Germany, reaching a total prescription count of over 6 million in 1995.[1] German
physicians consider ginkgo as effective as any drug treat-

ment for Alzheimer's disease and
other severe forms of memory
and mental function decline.
(For more information on the
use of ginkgo for mental function, see *The Natural Pharmacist
Guide to Ginkgo and Memory*.)

**A special extract of
ginkgo leaf is the
most widely pre-
scribed herb in
Germany.**

Ginkgo is widely used for ordinary, age-related memory loss as
well. Many women have tried it
for the much milder symptoms
that strike all of us as the decades
go on—such as walking into a room and forgetting why you
came in (wryly called "destinesia"), or being unable to recall a name that you remembered the day before.

Interestingly, some women who took ginkgo for this
purpose noticed an interesting "side effect." The fluid
buildup that they were accustomed to experiencing each
menstrual cycle seemed to diminish. They felt more comfortable, free of that heavy, waterlogged sensation. Reports of experiences such as these eventually led to a
formal study of ginkgo as a treatment for PMS-related
fluid retention.

What Is the Scientific Evidence for Ginkgo?

In 1993, two French researchers published the results of a
double-blind study that found ginkgo effective for the
treatment of "congestive symptoms" related to PMS.[2] By
this term they meant all the symptoms of fluid retention,
including breast tenderness and pain, abdominal or pelvic
pain and swelling, and swollen extremities—hands, fingers, legs, and feet. They also examined its effect on other

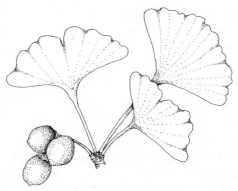

Figure 7. *Ginkgo*

PMS symptoms that they felt might be related to fluid buildup, such as headache and irritability.

The study evaluated 143 women, 18 to 45 years of age, and followed them for two menstrual cycles. All women admitted to the study had experienced PMS-related congestive symptoms for at least three consecutive cycles. When the study began, each woman received either ginkgo extract or placebo on day 16 of the first cycle. Treatment was continued until day 5 of the next cycle, and resumed again on day 16 of that cycle.

The results were impressive. As compared to placebo, ginkgo significantly relieved major symptoms of fluid accumulation, especially breast pain.

Although this was only one study, it was reasonably large,

As compared to placebo, ginkgo significantly relieved major symptoms of fluid accumulation, especially breast pain.

and the results deserve to be taken seriously. If additional research confirms these results, ginkgo may soon become widely accepted as a treatment for PMS.

Dosage

You can't simply grab a handful of ginkgo leaves, boil them in water, and expect to achieve the same results seen in the study I just described. The form of ginkgo used in this and all other scientific studies is a highly concentrated extract, in which 50 pounds of the leaf must be used to create 1 pound of product. Such extracts are standardized to contain 24% by weight of substances known as ginkgo flavonol glycosides. The proper dosage of ginkgo is 40 to 80 mg 3 times daily. It should be taken from about 2 weeks prior to your menstrual period until bleeding stops.

Safety Issues

Ginkgo extract appears to be quite safe. A review of nearly 10,000 participants taking ginkgo extract showed that less than 1% experienced side effects, and those that did occur were minor.[3] In another study, overall side effects were no greater in the ginkgo group than in the placebo group.[4] When a medication produces no more side effects than the placebo, we can reasonably regard it as essentially side-effect free. Furthermore, according to animal studies, ginkgo is safe even when taken in massive overdose.[5]

However, taking ginkgo presents one potential concern. The herb possesses a mild blood-thinning effect that could conceivably cause bleeding problems in certain situations. For this reason, people with hemophilia should not take ginkgo except on a physician's advice. Using ginkgo in the weeks prior to or just after major surgery or labor and delivery is also not advisable. Finally, ginkgo should not be combined with blood-thinning drugs such as Coumadin (warfarin), heparin, aspirin, and Trental (pentoxifylline), except under medical supervision. Ginkgo might also conceivably interact with natural products that slightly thin the blood as well, such as garlic and high-dose vitamin E.

The safety of ginkgo for young children, pregnant or nursing women, or people with kidney or liver disease has not been established.

Black Cohosh: Mainly for Menopause, but Might Work for PMS

Black cohosh (*Cimicifuga racemosa*) is a tall perennial herb that grows abundantly in North America, from Canada to the southern United States (see figure 8). The blackish, cylindrical root of this plant is the part used as an herbal remedy and perhaps is what gives this herb its name.

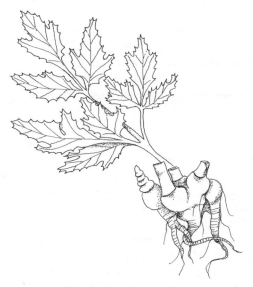

Figure 8. *Black cohosh*

Black cohosh is most famous as a treatment for menopause. It appears to produce an estrogen-like effect and thereby reduce symptoms, such as hot flashes and vaginal dryness.[6,7,8] (See *The Natural Pharmacist Guide to Menopause* for more information on using black cohosh for menopausal symptoms.)

Black cohosh is widely used for PMS symptoms, but we have no evidence that it is effective.

Black cohosh is also widely used for PMS symptoms as well. According to some reports, it can sometimes reduce all major symptoms, including anxiety, irritability, fluid retention, and breast pain. Unfortunately, there is no scientific evidence that black cohosh is effective.

Dosage

Black cohosh is sold as a standardized extract that contains 1 mg of 27-deoxyacteine per tablet. The standard dosage is 1 or 2 tablets, twice daily. If you purchase black cohosh in another form or concentration, you should follow the directions on the label to determine proper dosage.

Safety Issues

Black cohosh appears to be quite safe. It seldom causes side effects other than mild digestive distress, and animal studies have found no significant toxicity even when black cohosh was given at 90 times the therapeutic dosage for a period of 6 months.[9] Since 6 months for a rat corresponds to decades for a human, this study appears to make a strong statement about the long-term safety of black cohosh. However, because of its apparent estrogen-like effects, we don't know whether it is safe for women who have had breast cancer to take black cohosh.

In certain animals, this herb has been found to slightly lower blood pressure and blood sugar.[10] Therefore, it is possible that this herb could interact with drugs for high blood pressure or diabetes, although such an occurrence hasn't been reported in people. Black cohosh also might conceivably interact with other hormonally active substances, such as birth control pills.

Pregnant or nursing women should not take black cohosh. Its safety in those with liver or kidney disorders is not known.

Be sure you don't mistake black cohosh for blue cohosh (*Caulophyllum thalictroides*), which contains substances that are toxic to the heart.

Dong Quai: Widely Recommended As a "Female Tonic"

Dong quai has been used for thousands of years in China, and is among the major herbs in the repertoire of Chinese herbalists (see figure 9). Medical practitioners often

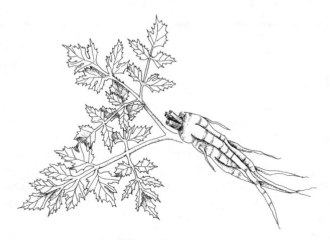

Figure 9. *Dong quai*

Anne's Story

Anne's PMS symptoms consisted primarily of irritability and moodiness. Her appetite also fluctuated dramatically, and she had back pain for 3 full days before menstruation started.

Since Anne was concerned that these symptoms might be a sign of serious medical problems, she went first to her gynecologist. After an examination, her doctor reassured her that she didn't have any condition that might be dangerous, and suggested antidepressant drugs for her symptoms. Anne, however, decided to experiment a bit first.

She visited a certified Chinese herbalist, who prescribed an herbal mixture containing dong quai as well as seven other herbs. The herbalist said that this formula should "harmonize her energy around the menstrual cycle." Anne, a skeptic about such things, thought his words sounded like mumbo-jumbo. Nonetheless, she decided to give it a try.

recommend dong quai as a treatment for PMS. However, no scientific evidence is available to support this use at this time.

Dong quai is the dried root of *Angelica sinensis,* a member of the parsley family. It is also closely related to the European *Angelica archangelica,* a common garden herb and the flavoring in Benedictine and Chartreuse liqueurs. Dong quai thrives in the high, cool mountain woodlands of southern and western China. Most of the world's supply of this herb is grown commercially, rather than harvested wild. The carrot-

Anne took 2½ teaspoons 3 times daily of a powdery medicine, making it into tea. After about 6 weeks of treatment, Anne noticed that her back no longer ached. Then another month passed and she found herself sailing smoothly through what was usually a rough premenstrual time, with no temper outbursts or crying spells. Her herbalist then changed the herb formula, and asked her to come back once a month. Each time Anne returned, he altered the herbal formula again, to help her "come in for a soft landing," as he put it. After a year, Anne has stopped taking the treatment altogether and none of the symptoms that had bothered her prior to treatment have returned.

Stories like these are intriguing and suggest that the complex techniques of Chinese herbal medicine should be investigated further. However, at the present time we have very little good scientific evidence regarding the effectiveness or safety of this ancient and traditional approach to healing.

like roots of this fragrant plant are harvested in the fall, after about 3 years of cultivation.

In the late 1800s, an extract of dong quai known as Eumenol became popular in Europe as a "female tonic." Today, dong quai is often recommended in the West as a treatment for PMS, as well as for menstrual cramps and menopause. However, in traditional Chinese medicine, the herb is not used this way at all. Rather than prescribing it alone as a one-size-fits-all PMS herb, properly trained Chinese herbalists combine it with other herbs to form a highly individualized treatment. (For more information on dong quai, see *The Natural Pharmacist: Your Complete Guide to Herbs.*)

Dosage

Using dong quai under the direction of a qualified Chinese herbalist may provide you with the greatest benefit. If you wish to treat yourself, a typical dosage is 10 to 40 drops of dong quai tincture 1 to 3 times daily. Since dong quai may be available in many forms and concentrations, I suggest that you follow the directions on your bottle of dong quai.

Safety Issues

Dong quai is believed to be generally nontoxic. Very large amounts have been given to rats without causing harm.[11] Side effects are rare and are primarily limited to mild digestive distress and occasional allergic reactions, such as a rash. Certain constituents of dong quai can cause increased sensitivity to sunlight, but this has not been observed in people using the whole herb.

Safety in young children, pregnant or nursing mothers, or those with liver or kidney disorders has not been established. Traditionally, the use of dong quai is prohibited during the first 3 months of pregnancy, for women with excessively heavy menstruation, or for individuals experiencing acute respiratory infections.

QUICK
REVIEW

- The herb ginkgo is most widely used as a treatment for impaired memory and mental function. However, a recent study suggests that it may help PMS symptoms as well, especially those related to fluid retention.

- The proper dosage of ginkgo is 40 to 80 mg 3 times daily of an extract standardized to contain 24% ginkgo flavonol glycosides.

- Ginkgo should not be taken by individuals with bleeding disorders such as hemophilia, combined with blood-thinning drugs, or taken during the period just before and after major surgery or labor and delivery, except under medical supervision.

- The herb black cohosh is widely used for menopausal symptoms, but it may be helpful for PMS as well. Standard dosage is 1 or 2 tablets twice daily of an extract containing 1 mg of 27-deoxyacteine per tablet.

- The Chinese herb dong quai (usually given in combination with other herbs) is also sometimes recommended for PMS. However, no studies as yet can document these potential uses.

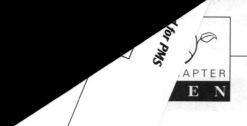

Herbs for PMS-Related Conditions

I f you suffer from PMS-related migraine headaches, your physician may prescribe a standard
antimigraine medication, even if that medication
has not been tested specifically in PMS. Similarly, several
herbs may be recommended for PMS because evidence
shows that they help with problems that occur in association with PMS. These herbs include St. John's wort for depression, kava for anxiety, and feverfew for migraines.

This chapter briefly introduces each of these interesting
and (at least in the case of St. John's wort) well-documented
herbs. For further information, see THE NATURAL PHARMA-
CIST series book devoted specifically to that herb.

St. John's Wort: A Well-Studied Herbal Treatment for Depression

If you are one of the many women who suffer from mild
depression during the premenstrual days of your monthly
cycle, take heart. St. John's wort, or *Hypericum perfora-*

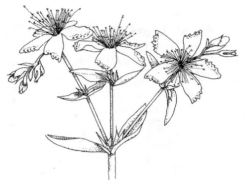

Figure 10. *St. John's wort*

tum, is a safe and mild herbal treatment that may be of benefit to you.

This common perennial herb of many branches and bright yellow flowers grows wild in much of the world (see figure 10). Its name derives from the herb's tendency to flower around the feast of St. John. (A "wort" is simply a plant in Old English.) The species name *perforatum* derives from the watermarking of translucent dots that can be seen when the leaf is held up to the sun.

St. John's wort is a scientifically well-established herbal treatment for mild to moderate depression.[1,2,3] It has been the number-one antidepressant used in Germany for some time, and recently achieved that status in the United States as well.

While no studies have yet evaluated the effects of St. John's wort on PMS, it seems logical that if this herb can relieve the symptoms of mild to moderate depression in general, it should be able to help similar symptoms associated with PMS. Keep in mind that standard antidepressants are prescribed for PMS based on the same principle.

What Is the Scientific Evidence for St. John's Wort?

St. John's wort is one of the best documented of all herbal treatments. According to a 1996 report published in the *British Medical Journal,* up to that time researchers had conducted 23 randomized, double-blind clinical trials of St. John's wort, enrolling a total of more than 1,700 participants.[4] The report suggested that the results made a compelling case for this traditional herbal remedy.

St. John's wort has been the number-one antidepressant used in Germany for some time, and recently achieved that status in the United States as well.

Since then, further studies have been performed. The best designed of these followed 147 people diagnosed with mild to moderate depression.[5] Its primary purpose was to determine whether a substance named hyperforin is one of the active ingredients in St. John's wort. Participants were given either placebo or one of two forms of St. John's wort: a low hyperforin product (0.5%) or a high hyperforin product (5%).

The results showed that the form of St. John's wort containing 5% hyperforin was successful in controlling symptoms of depression in about 50% of cases, a better result than placebo, while the low hyperforin product did not work. This suggests that hyperforin may be a major active ingredient in the herb. (For more information on St. John's wort, see *The Natural Pharmacist Guide to St. John's Wort and Depression.*)

Dosage

St. John's wort is available as a standardized extract, typically manufactured to contain 0.3% by weight of a substance named hypericin. However, based on the study just described, newer forms of the herbal extract are standardized to 3 to 5% hyperforin instead. Either way, the proper adult dosage of St. John's wort is 300 mg 3 times daily. Alternatively, you can divide the same daily dose into 2 rather than 3 parts. You will need to take St. John's wort for at least 4 to 6 weeks to discover whether it's going to work for you.

Safety Issues

St. John's wort is essentially side-effect free. In the extensive German experience with St. John's wort as a treatment for depression, there have been no published reports of serious adverse consequences from taking the herb alone, and even minor side effects are not common.[6,7] Furthermore, animal studies involving enormous doses for 26 weeks have not shown any serious toxicity.[8]

Cows and sheep grazing on St. John's wort have sometimes developed severe and even fatal sensitivity to the sun. However, this has never occurred in humans taking St. John's wort at normal dosages.[9] In one study, highly sun-sensitive people were given twice the normal dosage of the herb.[10] The results showed a mild but measurable increase in reaction to ultraviolet radiation. The moral of the story is that if you are especially sensitive to the sun, don't exceed the recommended dose of St. John's wort and continue to take your usual precautions against sunburn.

Nonetheless, there might be problems if you combine St. John's wort with other medications that cause increased sun sensitivity, such as sulfa drugs and the anti-inflammatory medication Feldene (piroxicam). In addition,

Kirstin's Story

Kirstin dreaded the week before her period. During that one week each month, Kirstin found herself looking at life as though she were at the bottom of a deep, dark well. Every task became a struggle, and she felt tearful and gloomy.

Kirstin finally broached the subject with her doctor, and received a prescription for Prozac. For the first 2 weeks she felt anxious and had trouble sleeping, but this side effect soon subsided. The next month was even better. "I used to know exactly when my period was around the corner, based on my mood," she commented. "But this time it came quietly, with no depression leading up to it."

However, a new side effect developed after a couple of months. Kirstin found herself unable to achieve orgasm. Her physician explained that this problem is fairly common with Prozac, although by no means universal, and that this particu-

the medications Prilosec (omeprazole) and Prevacid (lansoprazole) may increase the tendency of St. John's wort to cause photosensitivity.[11]

There are concerns that regular use of St. John's wort might also increase the risk of cataracts.[12] While this is preliminary information, it may make sense to wear sunglasses when outdoors if you are taking this herb on a long-term basis.

Some experts have warned for some time that combining St. John's wort with drugs in the Prozac family (SSRIs) might raise serotonin too much and cause a number of serious problems.[13,14] Recently, case reports of such events have begun to

lar side effect was one of the major reason...
ing this treatment. He suggested she switch to...
antidepressant.

But around this time Kirstin read an article describing St. John's wort. The pharmacist in her local drug store explained the proper dosage to her, and Kirstin decided to try it. However, he advised that she quit taking Prozac for a full 3 weeks first, to allow it to wash out of her system. Prozac lingers in the body for a long time, and it may not be safe to combine St. John's wort with standard antidepressants.

Kirstin had one very bad PMS week that reminded her how much the Prozac had helped. But by the time her next period came around, she had been taking St. John's wort long enough for it to work. It has continued to work, and Kirstin no longer dreads that one particular week out of each month.

trickle in. Therefore, do not combine St. John's wort with prescription antidepressants except on the specific advice of a physician. Since some antidepressants, such as Prozac, linger in the blood for quite some time, you also need to exercise caution when switching from a drug to St. John's wort.

Perhaps the biggest concern with St. John's wort is the possibility that it may decrease the effectiveness of various medications, including protease inhibitors (for HIV infection), cyclosporine (for organ transplants), digoxin (for heart disease), warfarin (a blood thinner), oral contraceptives, chemotherapy drugs, olanzapine or clozapine (for schizophrenia), and theophylline (for asthma).[15,16,17] Fur-

...y wort and one of
...and then stop taking
...may rise. This rise in
...certain circumstances.
...ad to catastrophic conse-
...vort appears to have caused
...t rejection by interfering with
...e. Also, many people with HIV
take ...the false belief that the herb will
fight the ...The unintended result may be to reduce the pote... standard AIDS drugs. In addition, the
herb might decrease the effectiveness of oral contraceptives, presenting a risk of pregnancy.

Safety in young children, pregnant or nursing women,
or those with severe liver or kidney disease has not been
established.

Kava: Anxiety Relief

If you are experiencing anxiety and nervousness as part of
your PMS, kava may be just the thing for you (see figure 11).
Although the scientific evidence for kava is not as strong as is
that for St. John's wort, studies tell us that kava can provide
relief from symptoms of anxiety. And the good news is that
kava appears to provide this benefit without the fatigue,
drowsiness, and mental impairment that often accompanies
conventional antianxiety medications.

Kava, or *Piper methysticum,* a member of the pepper
family, has been cultivated and used for centuries by Pacific
Islanders as a ceremonial beverage. Captain James Cook, on
his celebrated voyages through the South Seas, reported how
village elders and chieftains would begin special meetings
with elaborate kava ceremonies. Typically, each participant
would drink 2 or 3 bowls of the chewed-up kava and coconut
milk. Kava was also consumed in less formal settings as a
mild intoxicant, as it seems to have a relaxing effect.

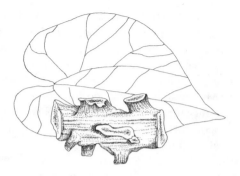

Figure 11. *Kava leaf and root*

When European scientists learned about the effects of kava, they set about trying to isolate its active ingredients. Although herbal products made from kava became available in Europe in the 1860s, it wasn't until 1966 that the substances known as *kavalactones* were discovered. One of the most active of these kava compounds is dihydrokavain, which has been found to produce sedative, painkilling, and anticonvulsant effects.[18,19,20]

Although no research has been performed specifically on women suffering from premenstrual syndrome, several double-blind studies document kava's effectiveness in the treatment of anxiety in general. It seems logical to believe that kava may also benefit those anxieties associated with PMS. (For more information on kava, see *The Natural Pharmacist Guide to Kava and Anxiety.*)

What Is the Scientific Evidence for Kava?

Researchers have conducted five meaningful studies of kava, involving a total of about 400 participants. The results show that kava can significantly decrease anxiety levels. However, some confusion remains about how rapidly it works.

The best of the studies was a 6-month double-blind trial that tested kava's effectiveness in 100 participants who exhibited various forms of anxiety.[21] Over the course of the trial, researchers evaluated each participant using a list of questions called the Hamilton Anxiety Scale (HAM-A). The HAM-A assigns a total score based on such symptoms as restlessness, nervousness, heart palpitations, stomach discomfort, dizziness, and chest pain. Lower scores indicate reduced anxiety.

The results showed that participants given kava showed significantly improved scores beginning at 8 weeks and continuing throughout the duration of the treatment.

Strangely, previous studies showed a good response in 1 week.[22,23,24] The reason why kava took so long to work in this one study remains unclear.

Dosage

Kava is usually sold in a standardized form for which the total amount of kavalactones per pill is listed. For use as an antianxiety agent, the dose of kava should supply about 40 to 70 mg of kavalactones to be taken 3 times daily. The total daily dosage should not exceed 300 mg of kavalactones. You will usually notice some improvement in a week or so, but results may take 4 weeks to develop fully.

Safety

When used appropriately, kava appears to be safe. Animal studies have found that dosages of up to 4 times the normal dose cause no problems at all, and 13 times the normal dosage causes only mild problems in rats.[25] Large studies designed specifically to look at side effects found no problems other than occasional mild digestive distress or allergic rashes.[26] However, long-term use (months to years) of kava in excessive doses (over 400 mg kavalactones daily) can create a distinctive generalized dry, scaly rash,[27] which disappears promptly when you stop taking kava.

Kava does not appear to produce mental cloudiness.[28,29,30] Nonetheless, I wouldn't recommend driving after using kava until you discover how strongly it affects you. It makes some people quite drowsy.

Safety in young children, pregnant or nursing women, or those with severe liver or kidney disease has not been established.

Warning: Kava should not be combined with alcohol, prescription tranquilizers or sedatives, or other depressant drugs. There has been at least one report of coma apparently caused by combining kava with prescription tranquilizers.[31]

Feverfew: A General Preventive Treatment for Migraines

Many women experience migraine headaches during PMS. While it hasn't been tested specifically for PMS migraines, the herb feverfew (*Tanacetum parthenium*) is widely used in the United Kingdom as a general preventive treatment for migraine headaches. It certainly seems logical to try it for PMS headaches as well.

Originally native to the Balkans, this relative of the common daisy was spread by deliberate planting throughout Europe and the Americas. Feverfew's feathery and aromatic leaves (see figure 12) have long been used medicinally to improve childbirth, promote menstruation, induce abortions, relieve rheumatic pain, and treat severe headaches.

The modern medical use of feverfew dates back to the late 1970s. At that time, the wife of the chief medical officer of the National Coal Board in England suffered from serious migraine

> **Feverfew is widely used in the United Kingdom as a general preventive treatment for migraine headaches.**

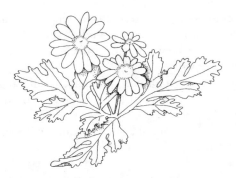

Figure 12. *Feverfew*

headaches. When workers in the industry learned of this fact, a sympathetic miner suggested she try a folk treatment he had used. She followed his advice and chewed feverfew leaves. The results were dramatic: Her migraines stopped coming.

Her husband was impressed, too. He used his high office to gain the ear of a physician who specialized in migraine headaches, Dr. E. Stewart Johnson of the London Migraine Clinic. Johnson subsequently tried feverfew on 10 of his patients. The results were so good that he subsequently gave the herb to 270 of his patients. A whopping 70% reported considerable relief.

Thoroughly excited now, Dr. Johnson enrolled 17 feverfew-using patients in an interesting type of double-blind study: Half were continued on feverfew and the other half were transferred, without their knowledge, to placebo.[32] Over a period of 6 months, the patients withdrawn from feverfew demonstrated a dramatic increase in headaches, nausea, and vomiting.

This preliminary study brought a flood of response from the public, and ultimately led to the properly performed double-blind experiments described in the following section.

What Is the Scientific Evidence for Feverfew?

Three double-blind studies have been performed to evaluate feverfew's effectiveness as a preventive treatment for migraines. Two returned positive results, the other negative. Based on these results, it seems that while feverfew leaf is effective, alcohol extracts made from feverfew may not work.

The Nottingham trial followed 59 participants for 8 months.[33] For 4 months, half received a daily capsule of powdered whole feverfew leaf; the other half was given placebo. The groups were then switched and followed for an additional 4 months. Treatment with feverfew produced a 24% reduction in the number of migraines and a significant decrease in nausea and vomiting during the headaches.

A recent Israeli study of 57 people with migraine who were given powdered feverfew leaf found a significant decrease in severity of their headaches.[34] Unfortunately, the study did not report whether participants experienced any change in the frequency of their migraines.

However, a Dutch study of 50 participants showed no difference whatsoever between placebo and a special alcohol-based feverfew extract standardized to parthenolide content.[35] Parthenolide is a substance that many had assumed was the

Feverfew has long been used medicinally to improve childbirth, promote menstruation, induce abortions, relieve rheumatic pain, and treat severe headaches.

active ingredient in feverfew. Apparently, this assumption was wrong, as this high-parthenolide extract did not work. The moral of the story is that if you take feverfew, you should stick to the leaf itself. (For more information on feverfew, see *The Natural Pharmacist Guide to Feverfew and Migraines.*)

Dosage

The usual recommended dosage of feverfew is 80 to 100 mg daily of powdered whole feverfew leaf. In contrast to most other herbs described in this chapter, no standardized extract is yet available that is known to work.

Feverfew is also sometimes taken at the onset of a migraine headache to reduce symptoms.

Safety Issues

Among the many thousands of people who use feverfew as a folk medicine in England, there have been no reports of serious toxicity. Furthermore, animal studies and the results of clinical trials in people suggest that feverfew is essentially nontoxic, although more study remains to be done.[36,37]

Feverfew seldom causes side effects other than occasional mild digestive distress.[38] However, if you chew feverfew leaf, rather than take it in capsules, you might develop mouth sores. In view of its use as a folk remedy to promote abortions, feverfew should probably not be taken during pregnancy. Safety in young children, pregnant or nursing women, or those with severe kidney or liver disease has not been established.

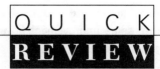

- St. John's wort is one of the best-documented of all herbal treatments. The results of numerous studies tell us that St. John's wort can provide relief for mild to moderate depression. Although no studies have focused on St. John's wort and PMS, it seems reasonable to think that the herb might also be effective for the symptoms of mild depression that accompany PMS.

- St. John's wort is available as a standardized extract, typically manufactured to contain 0.3% by weight of a substance named hypericin. Newer forms of the herbal extract are standardized to 3 to 5% hyperforin instead. Either way, the proper adult dosage of St. John's wort is 300 mg 3 times daily. Alternatively, you can divide the same daily dose into 2 rather than 3 parts. You will need to take St. John's wort for at least 4 to 6 weeks to discover whether it's going to work.

- St. John's wort should not be combined with prescription antidepressants, and for certain drugs, such as Prozac, doctors recommend a wash-out period of several weeks before starting the herb. Refer to earlier in the chapter for other safety issues.

- Kava appears to reduce anxiety symptoms, although again it has not been specifically tested in PMS.

- Kava is usually sold in a standardized form where the total amount of kavalactones per pill is listed. For use as an antianxiety agent, the dose of kava should supply about 40 to 70 mg of kavalactones to be taken 3 times daily. The total daily dosage should not exceed 300 mg of kavalactones. You will usually notice some improvement in a week or so, but full results may take 4 weeks to develop.

- Do not combine kava with alcohol, prescription tranquilizers or sedatives, or other depressant drugs, as such combinations have led to reports of coma. Refer to the chapter for more safety information.

- Feverfew is widely used in the United Kingdom to prevent migraines. The proper dosage is about 80 to 100 mg daily of powdered whole feverfew leaf.

CHAPTER
ELEVEN

Lifestyle Changes

W hile this book has concentrated on medications, herbs, and supplements up till now, I don't want to leave the impression that these are the only approaches to dealing with PMS. For all health problems, lifestyle issues must be considered along with specific treatments in order to improve symptoms and overall health. Many women report they are able to better manage their PMS by making dietary changes, exercising on a regular basis, and learning how to reduce stress. It certainly makes sense that a healthy, low-stress lifestyle will leave you feeling better during any time of your monthly cycle. This point of view is shared by many physicians, who frequently recommend these lifestyle changes to their patients.

This chapter will discuss some of the "whole person" steps you can take to improve your health.

Meghan's Story

Exercise directs my energy," says Meghan. "I'm a lot less apt to fly off the handle. All my adrenaline and pent-up hormones have somewhere to go!"

She also readily admits that exercise tends to make everything go more smoothly throughout the day. In Meghan's case, "everything" includes helping her mother with the daily care of her grandmother, who has Alzheimer's disease, and commuting an hour each way to work. Meghan's day also includes the smaller tasks of going to the post office, sorting through the mail, paying bills, and taking care of the minutiae of everyday life.

Exercise and PMS

Experience suggests that moderate exercise may be able to reduce and even prevent premenstrual symptoms.[1,2] Thirty minutes or more each day may be all the exercise you'll need to realize these benefits. Many women readily attest that a consistent, moderate exercise program helps reduce their PMS symptoms.

Why Exercise May Help with PMS

While no double-blind placebo-controlled scientific studies are available to prove the effects of exercise on PMS[3,4] (after all, how would researchers manage a placebo for exercise?), scientific reasons tell us that it makes sense. The most popular theory suggests that "feel good" brain chemicals, called *beta endorphins,* are released when we exercise.[5] Beta endorphins are substances that our bodies manufacture to relieve pain. Beta endorphins are also thought to be involved in controlling the body's response

As a customer service representative for a financial investment company, Meghan spends at least 8 hours a day in a chair with either a phone glued to her ear or her fingers rolling over a keyboard. "It's a very caged feeling," she says. "When I go home—well, if I have PMS and I haven't exercised, look out! I can explode from all the pressure that's been building all day!"

At the age of 23, she already has a set routine that takes her to the local fitness center 3 days a week, where she does aerobics. The rest of the week she takes walks during her lunch break.

to stress. These substances appear to have pain-relieving effects and may be responsible for what is known as "runner's high," the feeling of elation athletes sometimes experience at moments of great exertion. Although we still have much to discover about beta endorphins, researchers think these substances may alleviate pain and help promote a feeling of well-being.

Another theory that may explain why exercise may benefit those with PMS is that women who exercise are less likely to experience food cravings and more likely to eat sensibly. In any case, you can't help but benefit from regular exercise. It strengthens the cardiovascular system, helps more oxygen get

Experience suggests that moderate exercise may be able to reduce and even prevent premenstrual symptoms.

to the brain, increases metabolism, helps with digestion and elimination, and strengthens the entire body so that our muscles, bones, and joints work better for us.

As we get into shape, we feel a sense of well-being. Our energy levels increase, and we are more ready to face challenges and deal with the stresses of everyday life. Since so many PMS symptoms relate to fatigue and a generalized feeling of being unable to "rise to the occasion," this increased energy may be a major benefit of exercise on PMS.

Finding the Right Exercise Routine

What kind of exercise you choose is not important; what's important is taking the first step. Walking, jogging, cycling, and aerobics are all of relatively equal benefit. In-line skating, swimming, and dancing are just as useful. Trying something first that doesn't require a lot of equipment is probably a good idea. You'll find it easier and cheaper, and you can start sooner.

As we get into shape, our energy levels increase, and we are more ready to face challenges and deal with the stresses of everyday life.

No matter what activity you choose, be sure it's something you enjoy. Continuing a regular exercise routine is easier when you like what you're doing. If you don't like to feel sweaty, try swimming. If you hate working out alone, find a convenient aerobics class. Once you select an activity and establish a routine you enjoy, you'll find it much easier to exercise consistently.

Learning to Set Your Pace

When you start out, be careful not to overexert yourself. You will be more prone to injury and fatigue when you first begin to exercise, and overdoing it may deflate your enthusiasm. If you haven't exercised regularly for a long while, you may wish to check with your doctor to determine what exercise might be best for you. He or she may be able to assist you in structuring a suitable program, and help you recognize the signs of overexertion.

Many people start out by walking 30 minutes a day. Walking is a low-impact form of exercise. It's easy to schedule, and you don't have to drive to a gym or pay money for a class. You may not even have to shower afterward. Not only will walking improve your physical well-being, but it can also be a time for meditating or socializing. Whether you walk in groups or with a partner, walking can provide companionship, stimulating conversation, and interaction. Walking with your children or your husband can be an activity that nurtures your family and your relationships.

> **Walking, jogging, cycling, and aerobics are all of relatively equal benefit. In-line skating, swimming, and dancing are just as useful.**

Some women enjoy walking in neighborhood and community groups. Such activity not only helps you keep in touch with what's happening around you, but also can provide the moral support women with PMS especially seem to need. If you are meeting other people, you are more likely to make it to your daily "walk times." And if you are competitive by nature, walking with others who are similarly inclined may provide you with the challenge and stimulation you need to take exercise to the next level.

Exercise and Your PMS Diary

Do you remember the PMS diary we told you about in chapter 2? Now is an especially good time to use it. When

Wanda's Story

At age 35, Wanda was already starting to feel old. When she pushed her children in the stroller, she felt exhausted after a couple of blocks. She woke up tired and went to bed tired.

When her friend Laura suggested she exercise, Wanda threw up her hands. "I'm too tired to exercise," she said, practically crying. Laura agreed that it would be hard to start, but encouraged her to try.

"Once you get over the hump, things will improve," she promised. Tentatively, Wanda agreed to go for a walk with her friend every other day.

The first time they got together for exercise, Laura brought along a running stroller to replace the one Wanda typically

you begin your regular regimen of exercise, keeping track of what exercises you do along with what PMS symptoms you experience may be especially useful. Be sure to note if, for some reason, you are unable to do your day's exercise. You may find that after a few months of regular exercise, this diary may provide compelling evidence that exercise definitely eases your PMS symptoms.

Diet and PMS

Although no studies have investigated diet as a cause for PMS, experience suggests that some types of foods may affect the moods of premenstrual women more than other foods,[6,7,8] and shorter, 3-hour time intervals between meals may help relieve PMS symptoms.[9] This amounts to used. "I don't need it anymore," she explained. "You keep it for now." They walked briskly but didn't jog.

Wanda felt a little tired after the first day, but it wasn't bad at all. By the third week, she found herself looking forward to the next walk even before the day's walk ended. With Laura's encouragement, Wanda also began to eat more carefully. Eventually, they joined a yoga class where the participants took turns taking care of the children.

After 3 months Wanda took a look back and realized how far she had come. "How far?" she says. "About 10 years. I feel like I'm 25 again!" Good diet, exercise, and the company of friends are the best tonic.

the same simple, basic advice you've heard all your life: eat right and feel better.

This section is a guide to a generally healthful diet, along with specific suggestions for women with PMS. As with exercise, no double-blind studies are available to confirm or refute the effects of particular diets on PMS.

Living with Your Food Cravings

Many women experience peculiar appetite disturbances during the premenstrual days of their monthly cycles. For some women, it means having no appetite at all, but more commonly, it means experiencing strong desires for particular foods. The foods premenstrual women most commonly desire are sweetened carbohydrates such as cookies, pastries, or chocolate (in almost any form), and salty snack foods such as chips.

If you are driven by these intense food cravings, you probably know how hard it is to maintain a healthful diet when you're in the throes of PMS. You may even wonder what causes your peculiar urges. Do they result from a biological need for certain substances? Or are you simply feeling so bad that eating makes you feel better? (That we so seldom crave a salad or a piece of fruit might tell us something!)

The foods premenstrual women most commonly desire are sweetened carbohydrates such as cookies, pastries, or chocolate, and salty snack foods.

While little scientific knowledge is available to tell us *why* we get food cravings, we might better ask ourselves *what* a week or two of binge eating each month might be doing to our general well-being. (Despite what you may think when you're knee-deep in PMS, chocolate is *not* one of the essential food groups!)

The real concern is that the binge eating of PMS can lead to high intakes of fats and serious weight gain. Since we already know that a high-fat diet carries increased risk of heart disease, avoiding the unhealthy PMS-related urges would seem wise from that standpoint alone.

A 1987 study suggests that high-fat diets cause particular problems in PMS.[10] In this study, 30 women were put on a diet for 4 months, during which they derived 40% of their calories from fats. Afterward, they followed another 4-month diet in which they obtained only 20% of their calories from fats. Results comparing the two 4-month periods demonstrated that the tendency for bloating and for breast pain and enlargement was significantly lower with the 20% fat–calorie diet.

While most practitioners focus on helping women control their food cravings, some observe that, unless women consume what they crave, they become very irritable.[11] However, given that these high-fat foods are bad for our general health and that some evidence suggests a diet low in fats may actually help PMS, eating a more healthful diet would seem wise. A healthful diet *is* likely to make you feel better.

The key to maintaining a healthful diet and learning to live with your PMS food cravings is likely to be an approach that uses *moderation*. During PMS especially, keep to the basics of your healthful diet. If you happen to have food cravings, enjoy that chocolate truffle, but only on occasion.

The key to maintaining a healthful diet and learning to live with your PMS food cravings is an approach that uses *moderation*.

Eating Habits and the Food Pyramid

If good health can have a positive effect on premenstrual syndrome, then the eating habits of many people today probably promote PMS: eating on the run, skipping meals, and filling up on empty calories. Donuts, brownies, pastries, crackers, and carbonated beverages—all these "foods" give us the false sensation that we have met our dietary needs. In truth, our food choices may actually prevent us from getting what we really need from our diets— protein, vitamins, minerals, complex carbohydrates, and a proportionate percentage of dietary fat.

It is important not only to eat the right foods, but also to eat them in the proper balance. Again, moderation is the key. The USDA currently recommends 6 to 11 servings of bread, pasta, rice, or cereal; 3 to 5 servings of vegetables;

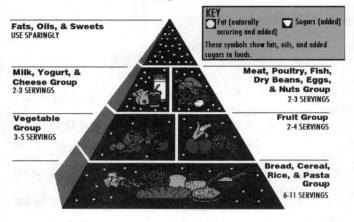

Figure 13. *Food pyramid recommended by the USDA*

2 to 4 servings of fruit; 2 to 3 servings of foods from the dairy group (milk, yogurt, cheese); 2 to 3 servings of meat, poultry, fish, dry beans, eggs, or nuts; and only small amounts of fats, oils, and sugary sweets (see figure 13). The ideal proportion of foods in your diet should be shaped like a pyramid with breads, pastas, and other grains at the base and fats and sweets at the top.

Unfortunately, our pyramids are often skewed and bloated. Instead of looking like the pyramid in figure 13, they may look more like figure 14. We may eat more fats and sweets than fruits and vegetables, and similarly, manage only minimal servings of milk and other dairy products. Such an unbalanced diet could lead to deficiencies of the vitamins, minerals, and nutrients that we need to maintain good health.

If your diet does not seem to be what it could be, don't worry; you can easily get on the right track by simply remembering these four general rules:

Typical Food Serving Pyramid

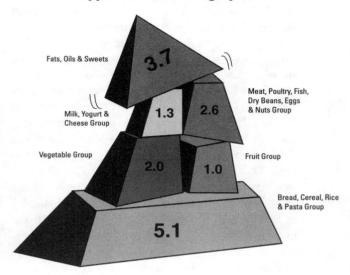

Figure 14. *Food pyramid showing the actual number of servings many people typically consume from each of the food groups.* (Adapted from the National Livestock and Meat Board and MRCA Information Services)

1. Drink 8 to 10 glasses of water or noncaffeinated beverage daily. Water is the most indispensable of all essential nutrients. In fact, by weight, our bodies are composed of about 60% water. Unlike solid food, which we can do without for long periods of time, we can only survive a few days without water.
2. Consume at least 5 servings of fruits or vegetables per day. The National Cancer Institute advises at least 5 servings of fruits or vegetables to help prevent cancer. (For more information on cancer prevention, see *The Natural Pharmacist Guide to*

Reducing Cancer Risk.) Fruits and vegetables also help prevent heart disease and many other illnesses as well. Besides vitamins and minerals, fruits and vegetables contain numerous other substances—such as flavonoids, carotenes, and sterols—that appear to improve overall health and prevent disease. You don't need these substances to live, but you may need them to live *well*.

3. Eat small meals and snacks frequently throughout the day. For many women with PMS, "3 squares a day" doesn't work. The answer may be "food grazing." This eating style incorporates 6 small meals into the day. The largest of these may be of the most benefit when eaten in the middle of the day or first thing in the morning. But don't forget to eat nutritious foods.[12] Try taking healthful snacks—such as fruit, yogurt, cartons of juice, whole grain muffins, rice crackers, and carrot sticks—to work.

4. Enjoy a diet rich in variety and strong in moderation. Each day, eat a variety of foods from all the essential food groups. If you eat meat, keep the portions small, balancing them with adequate quantities of grains and vegetables. Be sensible about the amount of fat that you consume.

Stress and PMS

Have you ever had the experience of knowing that you have to be in three places at once? Not just the "it's 3 o'clock and I'm still in traffic" sensation, but the "it's 3 o'clock and I'm still in traffic, and I'm 20 minutes late for my doctor's appointment (which I won't be able to reschedule for 6 months), and the post office will be closed when I get there so I can't mail the bill that was supposed to arrive 2 days ago, and why didn't I eat lunch" sensation? Well, this is stress.

There is no question that PMS involves stress. After all, one of its names is "premenstrual stress syndrome." It certainly stands to reason that reducing the stress in our lives and working to promote relaxation can have a positive effect on our PMS symptoms.

If you've ever wondered whether or not stress actually "triggers" your PMS symptoms, take a minute to look over the following list. Each item is loaded with stress, and depending on your response style, each can have a profound effect on your emotional well-being.

It stands to reason that reducing the stress in our lives and working to promote relaxation can have a positive effect on our PMS symptoms.

- New job or career
- Change in work hours
- Increase in responsibility (at home or work)
- Trouble with a superior
- Fired from job
- Death of a loved one
- Divorce or separation
- In-law trouble
- Marriage
- Reconciliation
- Birth or adoption of a child
- Award or professional recognition
- School (beginning or graduating)
- Illness or injury
- Taking care of parents
- Buying new home
- Moving or relocating
- Trouble with transportation
- Alcohol or drug dependency (yours or a family member's)

- Psychological, emotional, or physical abuse at home or work
- Sexual harassment
- Change in social activity
- Change in sleep patterns
- Change in eating habits
- Financial trouble
- Holidays and other social occasions
- Too many hours on the job or a stressful project

Now, when you simply *think* of these situations, where do you feel the stress? In your head? (Are your temples thumping?) In your chest? (Are you holding your breath?) These very important questions relate to your stress-coping styles. As you drive home from your doctor's appointment, are you humming along with the radio (having gotten past the day's frustrations), or are you still silently fuming, clutching the steering wheel, hunching over it with the proverbial dark cloud floating directly above your head?

Try to recognize when and where you feel the most tense and keep that in mind as you read about the following relaxation exercises.

Relaxation Techniques

If your PMS seems to go together with being "stressed out," then you may well benefit from one of these relaxation exercises. You can use these simple techniques to ease or control both your premenstrual symptoms and your reactions to them. Once you've read about each exercise, experiment with the ones that most interest you and that might fit best into your lifestyle.

Alternate Nostril Breathing

In India, this relaxation exercise is called *Pranayama,* or balanced breathing. It is easy to do at any time during the day and often provides immediate relief from stress.

Sit up straight, either cross-legged on the floor or in a chair. Don't extend your spine or stretch; instead, relax but keep your spine aligned. If you are in a chair, keep your feet flat on the floor. Close your eyes. Keep your elbow by your side while placing your right hand near your mouth.

Then, gently compress your right nostril with your index finger, and exhale slowly through your left nostril. Next, inhale slowly through your left nostril, squeeze your left nostril with the back of your index finger, and exhale through the right nostril. Then inhale through your right nostril and begin the pattern again. Keep your mouth closed throughout.

> ***Pranayama,* or balanced breathing, is easy to do at any time during the day and often provides immediate relief from stress.**

Follow this pattern for 5 minutes, keeping your breath slow and steady, and letting each inhalation and exhalation get longer as you feel more comfortable. Don't hyperventilate; just relax and breathe in and out.

When 5 minutes are up, or whenever you are ready, relax your hand, keep your eyes closed, and rest quietly for a minute or two before getting up. Pranayama helps you focus and relax your mind, and you can use it to calm anxiety attacks, break fits of uncontrollable sobbing, and soothe irrational anger.

Rhythmic Breathing

Rhythmic breathing is another easy meditative exercise you can do at any time to help calm your mind and ease anxiety. Lie down on your back on the floor. Put your hands on your upper abdomen so that you can feel your diaphragm move up and down as you breathe. Close your eyes and concentrate on your breathing. Inhale gently and deeply through the nose, counting slowly to six, and then exhale through the nose, again counting slowly to six. Let your breaths get longer as you relax, and focus your mind on your breathing, feeling it go in and out, and letting go of all other thoughts that arise. Focus only on your breathing. Relax your stomach, letting all the stress and tension in the stomach muscles dissolve.

Continue until you feel very relaxed.

Muscle Contraction Exercises

This exercise is useful for finding and releasing tension in your body. It is particularly useful if you tend to feel stress in specific areas of your body, such as in your shoulders or your jaw. (See Releasing Tension Traps for additional methods.)

Lie down on the floor, close your eyes, and breathe quietly for a minute or two. Then beginning with your feet, contract and release all of the muscles there, first clenching your toes tightly for a few moments and then letting them go. Do the same thing with your calves, your thighs, and your buttocks. Once you've finished with each body part, try not to move it. As you contract and release, imagine that you are actually getting rid of unwanted, tired energy. Expand your belly like a balloon and then let it out with a rush of air from your mouth; do the same thing with your chest. Clench and release your hands and then your arms. In succession, pull your shoulders up and release, down and release, back and release, and as if they would meet in front of your chest and release. Raise your head an eighth of an inch and then gently lower it back down. Open your mouth wide, stick out your tongue, and release. Scrunch up your face as tight as you can and release. Finally, imagine relaxing the muscles of your scalp and the top of your head.

When you are done, lie still and take stock of your body. If you feel any remaining tension, breathe into the area and relax it. Concentrate on your breath for a few moments, then gently move each part of your body, reawaken it, and get up.

Releasing Tension Traps

Most people have certain spots in which they typically "hold" tension (see figure 15). What this means is simply that when you get tense, a particular part of your body is most likely to

Just about any part of the body can be affected by stress.

react. Some people hold tension in their backs, others in their faces, and some people feel tension in their hands. Just about any part of the body can be affected by stress.

Below are various ways of working out tension in specific parts of your body. Check the following list for the areas where you store tension, and then consult the text descriptions that correlate to the numbers:

1. Head
2. Neck
3. Shoulders
4. Jaw
5. Upper back
6. Middle back
7. Lower back
8. Eyes
9. Arms
10. Stomach

For Stress in Areas 1, 2, and 3: For your head, neck, and shoulders, massage your head with both hands—gently so you don't pull your hair. This increases the circulation all over your scalp. Take a slow breath in and then let it out. Then gently let your head fall forward and begin a head rotation. Rotate your head over your right shoulder so it is parallel to the floor, and hold it there for 5 seconds. Then slowly roll your head so that it hangs loosely from the neck over your back, and again count to 5. Then roll your head

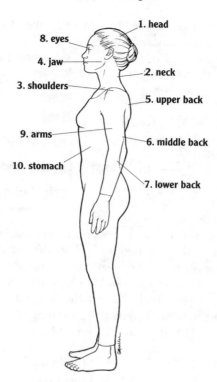

Figure 15. *Tension traps*

over your left shoulder and forward again. Repeat all these steps in the opposite direction.

For Stress in Area 4: To relax your jaw, open your mouth as wide as you can, then bring your lips together in the shape of an "O." Accentuate the movement of your lips as if you were shouting "Ow" in two elongated syllables. Say these syllables 25 times.

For Stress in Areas 5, 6, and 7: Several exercises can release tension in your back. First, stand with your feet comfortably apart and your arms comfortably at your sides, then take a breath and clasp your fingers behind your back. Exhale as you bend forward, bringing your clasped hands up and over your head. Hold this position for a few moments, relaxing further into the pose if you can do so without causing any pain. Exhale as you come back to standing position.

Second, with your feet comfortably apart, bend over, reaching for the floor with your fingertips, and touching it if you can. Let your head hang loosely; don't look at your hands. Then scoot your legs behind you until you can put the palms of your hands on the floor. Imagine that there is a string, or a rope, pulling you up by the small of your back toward the ceiling. Let it keep pulling you up. After about 5 seconds, let your back relax, bring your hands and feet closer together again, and stand. Repeat 3 times.

Third, standing with your feet comfortably apart, pick up your right leg and bend it toward your chest, clasping it lightly with your hands. Let go and pick up your other leg, bending it and clasping it toward your chest. Repeat, alternating legs, for 25 times each leg.

For Stress in Area 8: Most of us today spend prolonged periods of time staring at our computers and televisions, which are a predictable distance away, so it is important to stretch our vision. Look straight ahead for 2 seconds, preferably at something far away. Then look to the right for 2 seconds without turning your head. Look up for 2 seconds without turning your head. Look to the left for 2 seconds without turning your head. Repeat 3 times.

Apply cool gel packs, buckwheat husk eye pillows, or aromatherapeutic sachets when available or necessary. Cucumbers work wonders on the eyes. Peel them so they don't have skins, and put thin little slices on your closed lids.

For Stress in Area 9: To relieve stress in your arms, stand with your feet comfortably apart and rest your hands, one on top of the other, in the center of your chest. Your elbows should be perpendicular to the floor. Next, inhale deeply, and as you do, slide your hands up and toward your shoulders as your elbows move up and out. Hold this position for 5 seconds. Exhale. Repeat 3 times.

For the next exercise, rest your hands one over the other in the center of your chest. Inhale and throw them outward, as if you were gesturing in welcome, flinging your arms and hands away from your body as far as they will go. Bring them back to the chest in one fluid movement. Repeat 25 times.

Stand facing a wall, a little under arm's length away. Place your palms on the wall, and push your body away from it. Push and stretch as far as you can without actually moving away from the wall. Repeat 3 times.

For Stress in Area 10: Breathing meditations, done on your back, provide the best and most soothing relief to tense stomach muscles. Lie down and place your hands on your stomach. Breathe out slowly. With this exercise, be aware of what your stomach feels like when it is pressed out by your diaphragm. Now breathe in fully and try not to disturb that relaxed, extended pose by automatically contracting your stomach muscles when you breathe out. Imagine that you are releasing your stomach muscles, letting them go, and loosening them.

QUICK REVIEW

- Many women report that they are able to better manage their PMS symptoms by improving diet, exercising on a regular basis, and working to reduce the effects of stress in their lives.

- Exercise may relieve PMS symptoms by promoting the release of beta endorphins, natural chemicals that give a sense of well-being.

- It is important to exercise regularly, but you need to find the right kinds of exercises for yourself and to learn to set a pace that is comfortable, beneficial, and does not result in over-exertion.

- Eating a diet low in fat may provide some relief from the symptoms of PMS.

- By learning to reduce stress and to promote relaxation, you may be able to feel better throughout your menstrual cycle.

- Relaxation techniques that may help you reduce the effects of stress in your life include alternate nostril breathing, rhythmic breathing, muscle contraction exercises, and techniques for releasing tension traps.

CHAPTER
TWELVE

Putting It All Together

For your easy reference, this chapter contains a brief summary of key information contained in this book. Please refer to earlier chapters for more comprehensive information, including a detailed discussion of safety issues.

PMS is a monthly disorder with a number of symptoms that can cause significant annoyance and discomfort. We don't know as yet the cause of PMS or why some women are affected by it and others are not. There are a number of possible treatments for your symptoms, however. Conventional approaches include antidepressants, hormone therapies, antianxiety drugs, diuretics, and headache medications. You also have an assortment of natural treatments that may provide you with welcome relief from the various emotional and physical symptoms of PMS.

Natural Treatments for PMS

Recent evidence from a large double-blind study suggests that regular use of **calcium supplements** can dramatically reduce a wide variety of PMS symptoms, including depression, anxiety, crying spells, breast pain, bloating, food cravings, headaches, and general aches and pains. The suggested dosage is 1,200 mg of calcium daily.

The herb **chasteberry,** also known as vitex or *Vitex agnus-castus,* is widely used in Germany to treat the symptoms of PMS. The proper dosage of chasteberry varies with specific products. Chasteberry seldom causes any apparent side effects, but researchers have not yet performed full formal safety studies, so it should not be used by pregnant or nursing women.

Evening primrose oil has become an accepted treatment for the breast pain that often occurs in PMS known as *cyclic mastalgia.* The proper dosage is 2 to 4 g daily, taken with food. Evening primrose oil is safe and appears to be free of significant side effects; however, it works very slowly.

A recent study suggests that the herb **ginkgo** can help PMS-related fluid retention and breast tenderness. The proper dose is 40 to 80 mg, taken 3 times daily, of an extract standardized to contain 24% ginkgo flavonol glycosides.

Ginkgo appears to be quite safe, but there are some specific concerns about possible problems related to bleeding. For this reason, people with hemophilia should not take ginkgo except on a physician's advice. Using ginkgo in the weeks prior to or just after major surgery or labor and delivery is also not advisable. Finally, ginkgo should not be combined with blood-thinning drugs such as Coumadin (warfarin), heparin, aspirin, and Trental (pentoxifylline) except under medical supervision. Ginkgo might also conceivably interact with natural products that slightly thin the blood as well, such as garlic and high-dose vitamin E.

Other Possible Natural Treatments

Double-blind studies involving over 250 people suggest that **multivitamin/mineral tablets** can improve PMS symptoms (as well as your overall nutrition).

High doses of **vitamin E** may also reduce PMS symptoms. The recommended dosage is 400 IU daily; however, it should not be combined with blood-thinning substances such as Coumadin (warfarin), heparin, Trental (pentoxifylline), aspirin, garlic, or ginkgo except under medical supervision.

Some evidence suggests that **magnesium supplements** might improve PMS-related depression and symptoms of fluid retention. The usual dosage is 1,000 mg daily beginning on the 15th day of your menstrual cycle and continuing until the onset of your period. Magnesium at this dose is thought to be safe for healthy people, but if you have heart or kidney disease, do not use it (or any other supplement) except on medical advice.

Strong evidence tells us that the herb **St. John's wort** is helpful for depression in general, and as such might be worth trying for PMS depression. The proper dosage is 300 mg 3 times daily of an extract standardized to 0.3% hypericin or 3 to 5% hyperforin. If you decide to try St. John's wort but have been using certain drugs, such as Prozac, you will need to wait for some weeks after you stop taking the drug before taking the herb. Consult with your physician to determine the appropriate length of time.

Some evidence indicates that the herb **kava** can reduce anxiety symptoms in general, which suggests that it might be helpful for PMS-related anxiety. The proper dose should supply 40 to 70 mg of kavalactones to be taken 3 times daily. Kava should not be combined with alcohol, prescription tranquilizers or sedatives, or other sleep-inducing drugs.

The herb **feverfew** is widely used in the United Kingdom to prevent migraines and may be useful for menstrual migraines as well. The proper dosage is 80 to 100 mg daily of powdered whole feverfew leaf.

High doses of vitamin B_6 are often recommended for PMS symptoms, but studies have not found it to be effective.

Other herbs sometimes recommended for PMS symptoms include black cohosh and dong quai. However, there is no evidence as yet that they offer any benefit.

Stress reduction and a balanced diet may not only help PMS symptoms but also help your overall health.

Notes

Chapter Three

1. Thys-Jacobs S, et al. Calcium carbonate and the premenstrual syndrome: Effects on premenstrual and menstrual symptoms. *Am J Obstet Gynecol* 179(2): 444–452, 1998.

2. Werbach, M. Nutritional influences on illness, 2nd ed. Tarzana, CA: Third Line Press, 1993: 672.

3. Thys-Jacobs S, et al. 1998.

4. Borer M and Bhanot V. Hyperparathyroidism: Neuropsychiatric manifestations. *Psychosomatics* 26: 597–601, 1985.

5. Rojansky N, et al. Imipramine receptor binding and serotonin uptake in platelets of women with premenstrual changes. *Gynecol Obstet Invest* 31(3): 146–152, 1991.

6. Lee SJ and Kanis JA. An association between osteoporosis and premenstrual and postmenstrual symptoms. *Bone Miner* 24:127–134, 1994.

7. Thys-Jacobs S, et al. 1998.

8. Wang M, et al. Relationship between symptom severity and steroid variation in women with premenstrual syndrome: Study on serum pregnenolone, pregnenolone sulfate, 5-alpha pregnane-3, 20-dione and 3-alpha-hydroxy-5-alpha-pregnan-20-one. *Clin Endocrinol Metab* 81(3): 1076–1082, 1996.

9. Barrett-Connor E. Rethinking the estrogen and the brain. *J Amer Geriatr Soc* 46(7): 918–920, 1998.

10. Fink G, Sumner BE, Rosie R, et al. Estrogen control of central neurotransmission: Effect on mood, mental state, and memory. *Cell Mol Neurobiol* 16(3): 325–344, 1996.

11. Schneider H and Bohnet H. Hyperprolactinaemia and ovarian insufficiency. *Gynecology* 14: 104–118, 1981.

12. Lauritzen CH, et al. Treatment of premenstrual tension syndrome with *Vitex agnus-castus*. *Phytomedicine* 4(3): 183–189, 1997.

13. Horrobin DF, et al. Abnormalities in plasma essential fatty acid levels in women with premenstrual syndrome and with non-malignant breast disease. *J Nutr Med* 2: 259–264, 1991.

14. Horrobin DF and Manku MS. Premenstrual syndrome and premenstrual breast pain (cyclical mastalgia): Disorders of essential fatty acid (EFA) metabolism. *Prostaglandins Leukot Essent Fatty Acids* 37: 255–261, 1989.

15. Rapkin AJ, Morgan M, Goldman L, et al. Progesterone metabolite allopregnanolone in women with premenstrual syndrome. *Obstet Gynecol* 90(5): 709–714, 1997.

16. Smith SS, Gong QH, Hsu FC, et al. GABA(A) receptor alpha-4 subunit suppression prevents withdrawal properties of an endogenous steroid. *Nature* 392(6679): 926–930, 1998.

17. Dittmar FW, et al. Premenstrual syndrome. Treatment with a phytopharmaceutical. *Therapiewoche Gynakol* 5: 60–68, 1992.

Chapter Four

1. Mortola JF. A risk-benefit appraisal of drugs used in the management of premenstrual syndrome. *Drug Safety* 10(2): 160–169, 1994.

2. Stone AB, Pearlstein TB, and Brown WA. Fluoxetine in the treatment of late luteal phase dysphoric disorder. *J Clin Psychiatry* 52: 290–293, 1991.

3. Wood SH, Mortola JF, Chan YF, et al. Treatment of premenstrual syndrome with fluoxetine: A double-blind placebo-controlled crossover study. *Obstet Gyn* 80(3): 339–344, 1992.

4. Elks ML. Open trial of fluoxetine therapy for premenstrual syndrome. *South Med J* 86: 503–507, 1993.

5. Ozeren S, Corakci A, Yucesoy L, et al. Fluoxetine in the treatment of premenstrual syndrome. *Eur J Obstet Gynecol Reprod Biol* 73(2): 167–170, 1997.

6. Menkes DB, Taghavi E, Mason PA, et al. Fluoxetine treatment of severe premenstrual syndrome. *BMJ* 305: 346–347, 1992.

7. Brandenburg S, Tuynman-Qua H, Verheij R, et al. Treatment of premenstrual syndrome with fluoxetine: An open study. *Int Clin Psychopharmacol* 8: 315–317, 1993.

8. Pearlstein TB and Stone AB. Long-term fluoxetine treatment of late luteal phase dysphoric disorder. *J Clin Psych* 55(8): 332–335, 1994.

9. Steiner M, Steinberg S, Stewart D, et al. Fluoxetine in the treatment of premenstrual dysphoria. *N Engl J Med* 332(23): 1995.

10. Gunasekara NS, Noble S, and Benfield P. Paroxetine: An update of its pharmacology and therapeutic use in depression and a review of its use in other disorders. *Drugs* 55(1): 85–120, 1998.

11. Yonkers KA, Halbreich U, Freeman EW, et al. Sertraline in the treatment of premenstrual dysphoric disorder. *Psychopharmacol Bull* 32: 41–46, 1996.

12. Eriksson E, Hedberg MA, Andersch B, et al. The serotonin-reuptake inhibitor paroxetin is superior to the noradrenaline-reuptake inhibitor maprotiline in the treatment of premenstrual syndrome: A placebo-controlled trial. *Neuropsycopharmacology* 12: 167–176, 1995.

13. Pearlstein TB and Stone AB. 1994.

14. Steiner M, Korzekwa M, Lamont J, et al. Intermittent fluoxetine dosing in the treatment of women with premenstrual dysphoria. *Psychopharmacol Bull* 33(4): 771–774, 1997.

15. Balon R et al. Sexual dysfunction during antidepressant treatment. *J Clin Psych* 54: 209–212, 1993.

16. Graham CA and Sherwin BB. A prospective treatment study of premenstrual symptoms using a triphasic oral contraceptive. *J Psychosom Res* 36: 3257–3266, 1992.

17. Backstrom T, Hansson-Malmstrom Y, Lindhe BA, et al. Oral contraceptives in premenstrual syndrome: A randomised comparison of triphasic and monophasic preparations. *Contraception* 46: 253–268, 1992.

18. Freeman EW, Rickels K, and Sondheimer MP. A double-blind trial of oral progesterone, alprazolam, and placebo in treatment of severe premenstrual syndrome. *JAMA* 274(1): 51–57, 1995.

19. Vanselow W. Effect of progesterone and its 5 alpha and 5 beta metabolites on symptoms of premenstrual syndrome according to route of administration. *J Psychosom Obstet Gynaecol* 17(1): 29–38, 1996.

20. Derzko CM. Role of danazol in relieving premenstrual syndrome. *J Reprod Med* 35(Suppl. 1): 97–102, 1990.

21. Hahn PM, van Vugt DA, and Reid RL. A randomized, placebo-controlled, crossover trial of danazol for the treatment of premenstrual syndrome. *Psychoneuroendocrinology* 20(2): 193–209, 1995.

22. Mortola J. From GnRH to SSRIs and beyond: Weighing the options for drug therapy in premenstrual syndrome. *Women's Health* 2(10): Medscape Inc., 1997.

23. Wang M, Hammarback S, Lindhe BA, et al. Treatment of premenstrual syndrome by spironolactone: A double-blind placebo-controlled study. *Acta Obstet Gynecol Scand* 74: 803–808, 1995.

24. Leira R, Suarez C, Castillo J, et al. Subcutaneous sumatriptan in the treatment of migraine attacks. An analysis of its long-term efficaciousness and tolerance. *Rev Neurol* 23(122): 752–755, 1995.

25. Lauritzen C, et al. Treatment of premenstrual tension syndrome with *Vitex agnus-castus*. Controlled, double-blind study versus pyridoxine. *Phytomedicine* 4(3): 183–189, 1997.

26. Nickel JC. Placebo therapy of benign prostatic hyperplasia: a 25-month study. *Br J Urol* 81: 383–387, 1998.

Chapter Five

1. Werbach, M. Nutritional influences on illness, 2nd ed. Tarzana, CA: Third Line Press, 1993: 672.

2. Thys-Jacobs S and Alvir J. Calcium regulating hormones across the menstrual cycle—evidence of secondary hyperparathyroidism in women with PMS. *J Clin Endocrinol Metab* 80: 2227–2232, 1995.

3. Thys-Jacobs S, et al. Calcium supplementation in premenstrual syndrome: A randomized crossover trial. *Gen Intern Med* 4: 183–189, 1989.

4. Penland JG and Johnson PE. Dietary calcium and manganese effects on menstrual cycle symptoms. *Am J Obstet Gynecol* 168: 1417–1423, 1993.

5. Lee SJ and Kanis JA. An association between osteoporosis and premenstrual and postmenstrual symptoms. *Bone Miner* 24: 127–134, 1994.

6. Thys-Jacobs S, et al. Reduced bone mass in women with premenstrual syndrome. *J Women's Health* 4: 161–168, 1995.

7. Thys-Jacobs S, et al. Calcium carbonate and the premenstrual syndrome: Effects on premenstrual and menstrual symptoms. *Am J Obstet Gynecol* 179(2): 444–452, 1998.

8. NIH Consensus Development Panel on Optimal Calcium Intake. *Nutrition* 11: 409–417, 1994.

9. Curhan GC, Willett WC, and Rimm EB. A prospective study of dietary calcium and supplemental calcium and other nutrients as factors affecting the risk of kidney stones in women. *Ann Int Med* 126: 497–504, 1997.

10. Curhan GC, Willett WC, and Rimm EB. A prospective study of dietary calcium and other nutrients and the risk of symptomatic kidney stones. *N Engl J Med* 328: 833–838, 1993.

Chapter Six

1. Jones WHS. Pliny: Natural history (A.D. 23–79). Cambridge: Harvard University Press, 1980.

2. Blumenthal M (ed). The German Commission E monographs, therapeutic guide to herbal medicines. Boston: The American Botanical Council and Integrative Medicine Communications, 1998.

3. Commission E monograph. *Agni Casti fructus* (chaste lamb fruits). *Bundesanzeiger* 90, 1985, replaced 1992.

4. Dittmar FW, et al. Premenstrual syndrome: Treatment with a pharmaceutical. *Therapiewoche Gynakol* 5: 60–68, 1992.

5. Peteres-Welte C, et al. Menstrual abnormalities and PMS: *Vitex agnus-castus. Therapiewoche Gynakol* 7: 49–52, 1993.

6. Lauritzen C, et al. Treatment of premenstrual tension syndrome with *Vitex agnus-castus:* Controlled double-blind study versus pyridoxine. *Phytomedicine* 4(3): 183–189, 1997.

7. Lauritzen C, et al. 1997.

8. Sliutz G, et al. *Agnus castus* extracts inhibit prolactin secretion of rat pituitary cells. *Horm Metab Res* 25: 253–255, 1993.

9. Jarry H, Leonhardt S, Wuttke W, et al. *Agnus castus* als dopaminerges Wirkprinzop in Mastodynon. *NZ Phytother* 12: 77–82, 1991.

10. Jarry H, Leonhardt S, Gorkow C, et al. In vitro prolactin but not LH and FSH release is inhibited by compounds in extracts of *agnus-castus:* direct evidence for a dopaminergic principle by the dopamine receptor assay. *Exp Clin Endocrinol* 102: 448–454, 1994.

11. Winterhoff H. Arzeipflanzen mit endokriner Wirksamkeit. *N Z Phytother* 14: 83–94, 1993.

12. Wuttke W, Gorkow C, and Jarry J. Dopaminergic compounds in *Vitex agnus castus.* As cited in Leow D and Rietbrock N, (eds.). Phytopharmaka in forschung und klinischer anwendung. Steinkopff Verlag, Darmstadt, 1995: 81–91.

13. Propping D, et al. Diagnosis and therapy of corpus luteum insufficiency in general practice. *Therapiewoche* 38: 2992–3001, 1988.

14. Milewicz A, et al. *Vitex agnus-castus* extract in the treatment of luteal phase defects due to latent hyperprolactinemia. Results of a randomized placebo-controlled double-blind study. *Arzneim Forsch* 43(7): 752–756, 1993.

15. Wollenweber E and Mann K. Flavonols from fruits of *agnus-castus. Planta Med* 48: 126–127, 1983.

16. Saden-Krehula M, et al. 4-3-ketosteroids in flowers and leaves of *Vitex agnus-castus. Planta Med* 56: 547, 1990.

17. Goerler K, et al. Iridoid derivatives from *Vitex agnus-castus. Planta Med* 6: 530–531, 1985.

18. Newall, C. Herbal medicines: A guide for health-care professionals. London: Pharmaceutical Press, 1996: 19.

19. Dittmar FW, et al. 1992.

20. Peteres-Welte C, et al. 1993.

21. Dittmar FW, et al. 1992.

22. Peteres-Welte C, et al. 1993.

23. Cahill DJ, et al. Multiple follicular development associated with herbal medicine. *Hum Reprod* 9(8): 1469–1470, 1994.

Chapter Seven

1. Pye JK, Mansel RE, and Hughes LE. Clinical experience of drug treatments for mastalgia. *Lancet* 2: 373–377, 1985.

2. Drug evaluations subscription, Vol II. Endocrine drugs 6. Chicago, Illinois: American Medical Association, 1991: 6.

3. Pye JK, Mansel RE, and Hughes LE. 1985.

4. McFayden J. Cyclical breast pain—Some observations and the difficulties in treatment. *Br J Clin Prac* 46(3): 161–164, 1992.

5. Pashby NL, Mansel RE, Hughes LE, et al. A clinical trial of evening primrose oil in mastalgia. *Br J Surg* 68: 801, 1981.

6. Budeiri D, et al. I. Evening primrose oil of value in the treatment of premenstrual syndrome? *Controlled Clin Trials* 17: 60–68, 1996.

7. Collins A, Cerin A, Coleman G, et al. Essential fatty acids in the treatment of premenstrual syndrome. *Obstet Gynecol* 81: 93–98, 1993.

8. Khoo SK, et al. Evening primrose oil and treatment of premenstrual syndrome. *Med J* 153: 189–192, 1990.

9. Ockerman PA, Bachrack I, Glans S, et al. Evening primrose oil as a treatment of premenstrual syndrome. *Rec Adv Clin Nutr* 2: 404–405, 1986.

10. Puolakka, J, Makarainen L, Viinikka L, et al. Biochemical and clinical effects of treating premenstrual syndrome with prostaglandin precursors. *J Rep Med* 30: 149–153, 1985.

11. Horrobin DF and Manku MS. Premenstrual syndrome and premenstrual breast pain: Disorders of essential fatty acid metabolism. *Prostaglandins Leukot Essent Fatty Acids: Reviews* 37: 255–261, 1989.

12. Horrobin DF. Nutritional and medical importance of gamma-linolenic acid. *Prog Lipid Res* 31: 163–194, 1992.

13. Horrobin DF, et al. Gamma-linolenic acid: An intermediate in essential fatty acid metabolism with potential as an ethical pharmaceutical and as a food. *Rev Contemp Pharmacother* 1: 1–45, 1990.

14. Horrobin DF. Essential fatty acids in the management of impaired nerve function in diabetes. *Diabetes* 46(Suppl. 2): S90–S93, 1997.

15. Horrobin DF. 1992.

16. Horrobin DF. 1990.

17. Horrobin DF. 1997.

18. Horrobin DF. The regulation of prostaglandin biosynthesis by the manipulation of essential fatty acid metabolism. *Rev Pure Appl Pharmacol* 4: 339–383, 1983.

Chapter Eight

1. Reynolds MA and London RS. Efficacy of a multivitamin/mineral supplement in the treatment of the premenstrual syndrome. Abstract. *J Am Coll Nutr* 7(5): 416, 1988.

2. Stewart A. Clinical and biochemical effects of nutritional supplementation on the premenstrual syndrome. *J Reprod Med* 32(6): 435–441, 1987.

3. Chakmakjian ZH, Higgins CE, and Abraham GE. The effect of a nutritional supplement, Optivite for Women, on premenstrual tension syndromes: II. Effect on symptomatology, using a double blind, cross-over design. *J Appl Nutr* 37(1): 12–17, 1985.

4. Goei GS and Abraham GE. Effect of a nutritional supplement, Optivite, on symptoms of premenstrual tension. *J Reprod Med* 28(8): 1983.

5. Stewart A. 1987.

6. London RS, Sundaram G, Manimekalai S, et al. The effect of alpha-tocopherol on premenstrual symptomatology: A double-blind study. II. Endocrine correlates. *J Am Coll Nutr* 3: 351, 1984.

7. London RS, Murphy L, Kitlowski KE, et al. Efficacy of alpha-tocopherol in the treatment of the premenstrual syndrome. *J Reprod Med* 32(6): 400–404, 1987.

8. London RS, Sundaram GS, Murphy L, et al. The effects of a-tocopherol on premenstrual symptomatology. *J Am Coll Nutr* 2: 115–122, 1983.

9. London RS, Sundaram GS, Murphy L, et al. 1983.

10. Murray M. Encyclopedia of nutritional supplements. Rocklin, CA: Prima Publishing, 1996: 174.

11. Flink BE. Magnesium deficiency—Etiology and clinical spectrum. *Acta Med Scand* 647: 185–197, 1981.

12. Wester PO. Magnesium. *Am J Clin Nutr* 45(Suppl. 5): 1305–1312, 1987.

13. Facchinetti F, Borella P, Sances G, et al. Oral magnesium successfully relieves premenstrual mood changes. *Obstet Gynecol* 78: 177–181, 1991.

14. Walker A, et al. *J Women's Health* 9: 1157–1165, 1998.

15. Peikert A, et al. Prophylaxis of migraine with oral magnesium: results from a prospective, multi-center, placebo-controlled and double-blind randomized study. *Cephalalgia* 6(4): 257–263, 1996.

16. Murray M. 1996.

17. Kant AK and Block G. Dietary vitamin B_6 intake and food sources in the U.S. population: NHANES II, 1976–1980. *Am J Clin Nutr* 52: 707–716, 1990.

18. van der Wielen, et al. Dietary intake of water soluble vitamins in elderly people living in a western society (1980–1993). *Nutr Res* 14(4): 605–638, 1994.

19. Albertson AM, et al. Nutrient intakes of 2- to 10 year-old American children: 10 year trends. *J Am Diet Assoc* 92(12): 1492–1496, 1992.

20. Diegoli MS, da Fonseca AM, Diegoli CA, et al. A double-blind trial of four medications to treat severe premenstrual syndrome. *Int J Gynaecol Obstet* 62: 63–67, 1998.

21. Kleijnen J, Gerben TR, and Knipschild P. Vitamin B_6 in the treatment of premenstrual syndrome—A review. *Br J Obstet Gynaecol* 98(3): 329–330, 1991.

22. Parry G and Bredesen DE. Sensory neuropathy with low-dose pyridoxine. *Neurology* 35: 1466–1468, 1985.

23. Waterstone JA, et al. Pyridoxine neuropathy. *Med Jaust* 146: 640–644, 1987.

24. Zempleni J. Pharmacokinetics of vitamin B_6 supplements in humans. *J Am Coll Nutr* 14: 579–586, 1995.

Chapter Nine

1. Schulz V, et al. Rational phytotherapy. New York: Springer-Verlag, 1998.

2. Tamborini A, et al. Value of standardized *Ginkgo biloba* extract in the management of congestive symptoms of premenstrual syndrome. *Rev Fr Gynecol Obstet* 88(7–9): 447–457, 1993.

3. De Feudis FV. *Ginkgo biloba* extract: Pharmacological activity and clinical applications. Paris: Elsevier, 1991: 143–146.

4. Kleijnen J and Knipschild P. *Ginkgo biloba* for cerebral insufficiency. *Br J Clin Pharamcol* 34: 352–358, 1992.

5. De Feudis FV. 1991.

6. Jarry H, et al. Studies on the endocrine effects of the contents of *Cimicifuga racemosa,* I: in vitro binding of compounds to estrogen receptors; II: influence on the serum concentration of pituitary hormone in ovariectomized rats. *Planta Med* 1: 49–49, 1985.

7. Duker E, et al. Effects of extracts from *Cimicifuga racemosa* on gonadotropin release in menopausal women and ovariectomized rats. *Planta Med* 57: 420–424, 1991.

8. Stoll W. Phytopharmacon influences atrophic vaginal epithelium. Double-blind study: *Cimicifuga* versus estrogenic substances. *Therapeuticum* 1: 23–31, 1987.

9. Korn WD. Six-month oral toxicity study with Remifemim-granulate in rats followed by an 8-week recovery period. Hannover, Germany: International Bioresearch, 1991.

10. Newall C. Herbal medicines, a guide for the health-care professional. London: Pharmaceutical Press, 1996: 80.

11. Zhu D. Dong quai. *Am J Clin Med* 90: 3–4, 117–125, 1987.

Chapter Ten

1. Ernst E. St. John's wort, an antidepressant? A systematic, criteria-based review. *Phytomedicine* 2(1): 67–71, 1995.

2. Linde K, et al. St. John's wort for depression—An overview and meta-analysis of randomized clinical trials. *BMJ* 313: 253–258, 1996.

3. Laakman G, et al. St. John's wort in mild to moderate depression: The relevance of hyperforin for the clinical efficacy. *Pharmacopsychiatry* 31(Suppl.): 54–59, 1998.

4. Linde K, et al. 1996.

5. Laakman G, et al. 1998.

6. Smet P and Nolen W. St. John's wort as an antidepressant. *BMJ* 3: 241–242, 1996.

7. Woelk H, et al. Benefits and risks of the hypericum extract LI 160: drug monitoring study with 3,250 patients. *J Geriatr Psychiatry Neurol* 7(Suppl. 1): S34–38, 1994.

8. Schulz V, et al. Rational phytotherapy. New York: Springer-Verlag, 1998: 56.

9. Seigers CP, et al. Phototoxicity caused by hypericum. *Nervenhielkunde* 12: 320–322, 1993.

10. Brockmuller J, et al. Hypericin and pseudohypericin: Pharmacokinetics and effects on photosensitivity in humans. *Pharmacopsychiatry* 30(Suppl. 2): 94–101, 1997.

11. Mirossay A, Mirossay L, Tothova J, et al. Potentiation of hypericin and hypocrellin-induced phototoxicity by omeprazole. *Phytomedicine* 6(5): 311–317, 1999.

12. Roberts J. Presentation at the 1999 Meeting of the American Society for Photobiology.

13. Muller WEG, et al. Effects of hypericum extract on the expression of serotonin receptors. *J Geriatr Psychiatry Neurol* 7(Suppl. 1): S63–S64, 1994.

14. Muller WE, et al. Hypericum extract (LI160) as an herbal antidepressant. *Pharmacopsychiatry* 30(Suppl. 2): 71–134, 1997.

15. Jobst KA, McIntyre M, St. George D, et al. Safety of St John's wort (*Hypericum perforatum*). *Lancet* 355(9203): 575, 2000.

16. Nebel A, Baker RK, and Kroll DJ. Potential metabolic interaction between theophylline and St. John's wort. Submitted to *Annals of Pharmacotherapy*, 1998.

17. Baker RK, Sampey B, and Kroll DJ. Catalytic inhibition of human DNA topoisomerase II alpha by hypericin, a naphthodianthone from St. John's wort *(Hypericum perforatum)*. Manuscript in preparation.

18. Meyer HJ, et al. Kawa-Pyrone-eine neuartige Substanzgruppe zentraler Muskelrelaxantien vom Typ des Mephenesins. *Klin Wsch* 44: 902–903, 1966.

19. Klohs MW, et al. A chemical and pharmacological investigation of *Piper methysticum* forst. *J Me Pharm Chem* 1: 95–103, 1959.

20. Bruggermann F, et al. Die analgetische Wirkung der Kawa-Inhaltsstoffe Dihydrokawain und Dihydromethysticin. *Arzneim Forsch* 13: 407–409, 1963.

21. Volz HP, et al. Kava-kava extract WS 1490 versus placebo in anxiety disorders—A randomized placebo-controlled 25-week outpatient trial. *Pharmacopsychiatry* 30(1): 1–5, 1997.

22. Kinzler E, et al. Effect of a special kava extract in patients with anxiety-, tension-, and excitation states of nonpsychotic genesis. Double-blind study with placebos over 4 weeks. *Arzneim Forsch* 41(6): 584–588, 1991.

23. Warnecke G, et al. Wirksamkeit von Kawa-Kawa-Extract beim klimakterischen Syndrom. *Z Phytother* 11: 81–86, 1990.

24. Warnecke G. Psychosomatic dysfunctions in the female climacteric. Clinical effectiveness and tolerance of kava extract WS 1490. *Fortsch Med* 109(4): 119–122, 1991.

25. Schulz V, et al. Rational phytotherapy. New York: Springer-Verlag, 1998: 68.

26. Schulz V, et al. 1998: 71.

27. Norton SA, et al. Kava dermopathy. *Am Acad Dermatol* 31(1): 89–97, 1994.

28. Munte TF, et al. Effects of oxazepam and an extract of kava roots *(Piper methysticum)* on event-related potentials in a word recognition task. *Neuropsychobiology* 27(1): 46–53, 1993.

29. Heinze HJ, et al. Pharmacopsychological effects of oxazepam and kava-extract in a visual search paradigm assessed with event-related potentials. *Pharmacopsychiatry* 27(6): 224–230, 1994.

30. Herberg KW. Effect of kava-special extract WS 1490 combined with ethyl alcohol on safety-relevant performance parameters. *Blutalkohol* 30(2): 96–105, 1993.

31. Almeida JC and Grimsley EW. Coma from the health food store: Interaction between kava and alprazolam. *Ann Intern Med* 125(11): 940–941, 1996.

32. Johnson ES, et al. Efficacy of feverfew as a prophylactic treatment of migraine. *BMJ* 291: 569–573, 1985.

33. Murphy JS, et al. Randomized, double-blind, placebo-controlled trial of feverfew in migraine prevention. *Lancet* 2(3): 189–192, 1988.

34. Palevitch DG, et al. Feverfew (*Tanacetum parthenium*) as a prophylactic treatment for migraine: A double-blind, placebo-controlled study. *Phyto Res* 11(7): 506–511, 1997.

35. De Weerdt CJ, et al. Herbal medicines in migraine prevention. Randomized double-blind placebo-controlled crossover trial of a feverfew preparation. *Phytomedicine* 3(3): 225–230, 1996.

36. Newall C, et al. Herbal medicines: A guide for health-care professionals. London: Pharmaceutical Press, 1996: 120.

37. Murphy JS, et al. 1988.

38. Johnson ES, et al. 1985.

Chapter Eleven

1. Campbell EM, et al. Premenstrual symptoms in general practice patients: Prevalence and treatment. *J Reprod Med* 42(10): 637–646, 1997.

2. Johnson WG, et al. Macronutrient intake, eating habits, and exercise as moderators of menstrual distress in healthy women. *Psychosom Med* 57(4): 324–330, 1995.

3. Mortola J. From GnRH to SSRIs and beyond: Weighing the options for drug therapy in premenstrual syndrome. *Women's Health* 2(10): Medscape Inc., 1997.

4. Pearlstein TB. Hormones and depression: What are the facts about premenstrual syndrome, menopause, and hormone replacement therapy? *Am J Obstet Gyne* 173(2): 1995.

5. Goldfarb AH and Jamurt AZ. Beta-endorphin response to exercise: An update. *Sports Med* 24(1): 8–16, 1997.

6. Kurzer MS. The many conflicting thoughts aired concerning the relationship between a woman's moods and her food mostly serve as a reminder for us to eat sensibly. *Nutr Rev* 55(7): 268–276, 1997.

7. Christensen AP and Oei TP. The efficacy of cognitive behaviour therapy in treating premenstrual dysphoric changes. *Journal of Affective Disorders* 33(1): 57–63, 1995.

8. Lark SM. PMS: Premenstrual syndrome self-help book. Berkeley, CA: Celestial Arts, 1993.

9. Fernstrom MH and Fernstrom JD. Brain tryptophan concentrations and serotonin synthesis remain responsive to food consumption after the ingestion of sequential meals. *Am J Clin Nutr* 61(2): 312–319, 1995.

10. Jones, DV. Influence of dietary fat on self-reported menstrual symptoms. *Physiol Behav* 40(4): 483–487, 1987.

11. Wurtman JJ, et al. Effect of nutrient intake on premenstrual depression. *Am J Obstet Gynecol* 16(5): 1228–1234, 1989.

12. Fernstrom MH and Fernstrom JD. 1995.

Index

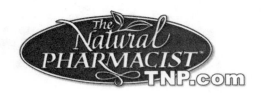

About the Author

Helen J. Batchelder has spent the past 5 years of her journalism career interpreting information relevant to the fields of medicine and phytochemical research. Currently a special projects writer for Integrative Medicine Communications (IMC) in Boston, Massachusetts, she has served as senior research editor for IMC, and was formerly the associate editor for Herbal Research Publications' Protocol Journal of Botanical Medicine.

About the Series Editors

Steven Bratman, M.D., medical director of Prima Health, has many years of experience in the alternative medicine field. A graduate of the University of California at Davis, Medical School, he has also trained in herbology, nutrition, Chinese medicine, and other alternative therapies, and has worked closely with a wide variety of alternative practitioners. He is the author of *The Natural Pharmacist: Your Complete Guide to Herbs* (Prima), *The Natural Pharmacist: Your Complete Guide to Illnesses and Their Natural Remedies* (Prima), *The Natural Pharmacist Guide to St. John's Wort and Depression* (Prima), *The Alternative Medicine Ratings Guide* (Prima), and *The Alternative Medicine Sourcebook* (Lowell House).

David J. Kroll, Ph.D., is a professor of pharmacology and toxicology at the University of Colorado School of Pharmacy and a consultant for pharmacists, physicians, and alternative practitioners on the indications and cautions for herbal medicine use. A graduate of both the University of Florida and the Philadelphia College of Pharmacy and Science, Dr. Kroll has lectured widely and has published articles in a number of medical journals, abstracts, and newsletters.